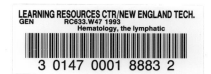

HEMATOLOGY, THE LYMPHATIC SYSTEM, AND THE IMMUNE SYSTEM

The REGENTS/PRENTICE HALL
MEDICAL ASSISTANT KIT

HEMATOLOGY, THE LYMPHATIC SYSTEM, AND THE IMMUNE SYSTEM

Third Edition

REGENTS/PRENTICE HALL, Englewood Cliffs, New Jersey 07632

Library of Congress Cataloging in Publication Data

Hematology, the lymphatic system, and the immune system. -- 3rd ed.
    p.   cm. -- (The Regents/Prentice-Hall medical assistant kit)
   Rev. ed. of: Hematology and the lymphatic and immune systems /
[Elizabeth K. White] 2nd ed. c1984.
   Includes index.
   ISBN 0-13-036690-0
   1. Blood--Diseases. 2. Lymphatics--Diseases. 3. Immunopathology.
4. Hematology.   I. White, Elizabeth K. Hematology and the
lymphatic and immune systems. II. Series.
    [DNLM: 1. Hematologic Diseases. 2. Immunologic Diseases.
3. Lymphatic Diseases.   WH 100 H487545]
RC633.W47 1992
616.1'5--dc20
DNLM/DLC
for Library of Congress   92-48846
                                              CIP

© 1993 by REGENTS/PRENTICE HALL
A division of Simon & Schuster
Englewood Cliffs, NJ 07632

Notice
The information and procedures described in the REGENTS/PRENTICE HALL MEDICAL
ASSISTANT KIT are based on consultation with practitioners and instructors and are to be
used as part of a formal course taught by a qualified Medical Assistant instructor. To the best of
the publisher's knowledge, this information reflects currently accepted practices; however, it
cannot be considered absolute recommendations. For individual application, the policies and
procedures of the institution or agency where the Medical Assistant is employed must be
reviewed and followed. The authors of these materials and their supplements disclaim responsibility for any adverse effects resulting directly or indirectly from the suggested procedures
and theory, from any undetected errors, or from the reader's misunderstanding of the materials. It is the reader's responsibility to stay informed of any new changes or recommendations
made by his or her employing health care institution or agency.

Printed in the United States of America

10   9   8   7   6   5   4   3   2   1

ISBN   0-13-036690-0

Prentice-Hall International (UK) Limited, *London*
Prentice-Hall of Australia, Pty Limited, *Sydney*
Prentice-Hall Canada, Inc., *Toronto*
Prentice-Hall Hispanoamericana, S.A., *Mexico*
Prentice-Hall of India Private Limited, *New Delhi*
Prentice-Hall of Japan, Inc., *Tokyo*
Simon & Schuster Asia Pte. Ltd., *Singapore*
Editora Prentice-Hall do Brasil, Ltda., *Rio de Janeiro*

Contents

Chapter 4. Diseases of the Lymphatic and Immune Systems

Preface

The REGENTS/PRENTICE HALL MEDICAL ASSISTANT KIT is the only textbook series written for students of Medical Assisting, which integrates the study of anatomy and physiology with diagnosis and treatment of disease. Our goal in this revision was to update and improve the series.

To achieve this goal, we solicited the advice of long-time users of the kit. Their comments resulted in many basic changes including simplification of concepts and procedures; addition of up-to-date information; an emphasis on quality control in all aspects of the physician's office laboratory; and enhanced study aids.

SIMPLIFICATION AND UP-TO-DATE INFORMATION

- All the books are infection-control–conscious throughout, reflecting the latest OSHA regulations.
- Anatomy and physiology titles have been simplified to reflect the very practical approach taken by many instructors.
- Diagnoses and treatments of disease have been updated for each body system.
- A thoroughly revised *Bio-Organization* launches the anatomy and physiology series with a simplified introduction to the structure and function of the body and a solid foundation for the study of human disease.
- *Laboratory Processes for Medical Assisting* is revised with more than 60 percent new material including performance-based procedure checklists for easy instructor evaluation, and the latest requirements of the Clinical Laboratory Improvement Act (CLIA).
- *Clinical Processes for Medical Assisting* now emphasizes only clinical procedures in the POL, leaving administrative issues to other more specific courses.

EMPHASIS ON QUALITY CONTROL

As the federal, state and local regulations become more specific, it is clear that the physician's major challenge is to provide not only the highest level of quality care and treatment for the patient, but also to document his or her commitment to that quality for the interest of government. It most often falls on the shoulders of the medical assistant to execute and police the quality control procedures within the office. The new laboratory books emphasize this need for quality control documentation.

The popular "Sources of Error" within the laboratory and clinical procedures checklists have been scrutinized and amplified.

ENHANCED STUDY AIDS

- Knowledge Objectives are grouped by chapter and by section.
- Pronunciations of medical terms are provided the first time a word is used. New terms appear in bold type and are defined in the extensive updated glossary.
- STOP AND REVIEW sections reflect Knowledge Objectives by section or by chapter.
- Over 60 new or revised illustrations and tables complement the text.
- All illustrations and tables are now precisely referenced in the text.
- Contemporary "sidebars" add spice and topical information to entice the student.
- Redesigned books emphasize organization and easy reading.
- Two new simplified four-color inserts are: A blood cell chart showing normal and abnormal blood cells; and 12 pages of body systems illustrations to accompany the *Bio-Organization* introduction.
- *Clinical Processes for Medical Assisting* includes the same type procedure checklist as *Laboratory Processes for Medical Assisting* for easy instructor evaluation.
- The laboratory books contain both Knowledge Objectives and Terminal Performance Objectives.

PREVIOUS BENEFITS RETAINED

The same strengths and benefits which instructors valued in the past have been retained or expanded:

- The flexible modular format can adjust to various program lengths or different orders of coverage for laboratory, clinical, and anatomy and physiology topics.
- The kit is written in a style specifically appropriate to the medical assisting student.
- The text/workbook style aids student learning. The material remains in small, manageable segments.
- The kit takes an integrated approach to structure, function, and disease of the human body.
- Each body system or medical specialty is followed by its clinical counterpoint of disease, diagnosis and treatment.
- A thorough review of disorders and diseases is classified by type in *Bio-Organization*, and by system through the subsequent anatomy and physiology 10-book series.
- The kit features an emphasis on quality control in *Laboratory Processes for Medical Assisting* and *Clinical Processes for Medical Assisting*.
- No prior knowledge of biology or chemistry is assumed.

ACKNOWLEDGMENTS

The revision of the Medical Assistant Kit represents a cooperative effort among many people. Foremost is Debra Grieneisen, M.T., C.M.A., who served as advisor for the series and in-depth reviser for *Laboratory Process for Medical Assisting*. Debra has taught medical assisting at Harrisburg Area Community College and Central Pennsylvania Business School, and it is her commitment to perfection that guided this work.

Several medical writers contributed to these books. Thank you to:

Karen Garloff, R.N.
Bruce Goldfarb
Steve Hulse
Ann Moy
Joy Nixon, R.N.

Cindy Jennings of BMR led the editorial efforts to manage this revision. Helping her were Nancy Priff and Rick Stull, as well as Jacqueline Flynn and Greg Flynn.

We particularly want to thank the reviewers whose advice, recommendations and collective knowledge helped form these books. Their concern for the subject matter, its accuracy, and primarily their students' best interest is reflected here. One thing they all agreed upon is the importance of accurate, clear illustrations which are integrated and referenced throughout the text. Our reviewers were:

Joanne Bakel
    Milton S. Hershey
    Medical Center
    Hershey, PA

Linda Barrer
    Lansdale Business School
    Lansdale, PA

Judy Bettinger
    Private Medical Practice
    Camp Hill, PA

C. Michael Cronin
    California College of
    Health Sciences
    National City, CA

Martha Faison
    Private Medical Practice
    Camp Hill, PA

Irene Figliolina
    Berdan Institute
    Totowa, NJ

Kathleen Hess
    Antonelli Medical &
    Professional Institute
    Pottstown, PA

Carol Kish
    Harrisburg Hospital
    Harrisburg, PA

Peter Kish
    Harrisburg Area
    Community College
    Harrisburg, PA

Tibby Loveman
    Gadsden Business College
    Gadsden, AL

Scott McKenzie
    Commonwealth College
    Virginia Beach, VA

Pat Morelli
    Medical Careers
    Training Center
    Ft. Collins, CO

Rhonda O'Grady
    The Laboratory Arts Institute
    Scarborough, Ontario

Sheila Ritchey
    Harrisburg Hospital
    Harrisburg, PA

Sandy Rishell
  Private Medical Practice
  Harrisburg, PA

Janet Sesser
  The Bryman School
  Phoenix, AZ

Shirley Seekford
  Antonelli Medical &
  Professional Institute
  Pottstown, PA

Robert Sheperd Kee
  Business College
  Norfolk, VA

Laura Silva
  The Sawyer School
  Pawtucket, RI

Pamela Smith
  Private Medical Practice
  Harrisburg, PA

Bruce Sundrud
  Harrisburg Area
  Community College
  Harrisburg, PA

Ann Sugarman
  Berdan Institute
  Totowa, NJ

Dan Tallman
  Northern State University
  Aberdeen, SD

Jackie Trentacosta
  Galen College
  Fresno, CA

Fred Ann Tull
  Southern Technical College
  Little Rick, AR

Deborah Wood
  Concorde Career Institute
  Lauderdale Lakes, FL

And finally, those who gave detailed feedback on our questionnaires helped configure the kit in its present form:

Theresa Bowser
  Southern Ohio College
  Columbus, OH

Elaine Chamberlin
  Pontiac Business Institute
  Oxford, MI

Thelma Clavon
  Rutledge College
  Columbia, SC

Leslie Fiore
  Kentucky College of Business
  Florence, KY

Diane Franks
  National Career College
  Tuscaloosa, AL

Tony Gabriel
  Watterson College
  Pasadena, CA

Karen Greer
  Sawyer College
  Merrillville, IN

Joyce Hill
  Lansdale School of Business
  North Wales, PA

Roxanne Hold
  Excel College of Medical Arts
  and Business
  Madison, TN

Annette Jordan
  Phillips Business College
  Lynchburg, VA

Martha Juenke
  American Medical
  Training Institute
  Miami, FL

Richard Krafcik
  Sawyer College
  Cleveland Heights, OH

Akeeboh Moore
  Career Com College
  of Business
  Oakland, CA

Basil Punsalan
  Commonwealth College
  Norfolk, VA

Alta Belle Roberts
  Metro Business College
  Rolla, MO

Sharon Adams
    Sasser Sawyer College
    Merrillville, IN
Joyce Shuey
    Academy of Medical Arts
    and Business
    Harrisburg, PA
Mary Ellen Stevenback
    Lansdale School of Business
    Harleysville, PA

Jinny Taylor
    Academy of Medical Arts
    and Business
    Harrisburg, PA
Edith Watts
    Watterson College
    Oxnard, CA

USING THE REVISED MEDICAL ASSISTANT KIT

The 10 anatomy and physiology books form the basis for a one-, two-, or three-term introduction to body structure and function and human disease. Each book stands alone and may be used in the most appropriate sequence for your program.

Laboratory Processes for Medical Assisting and *Clinical Processes for Medical Assisting* can supplement the anatomy and physiology books as lab sections or they can be offered as separate courses.

We hope instructors and students alike will find a certain new clarity and precision in this new edition of the REGENTS/PRENTICE HALL MEDICAL ASSISTANT KIT. We look forward to your comments.

Mark Hartman
Editor, Health Professions

The Language of Medicine

As you have studied the other books in this series, you have learned many Greek and Latin word parts, and have seen how they are put together to make words in the language of medicine. Now you need practice in putting those parts together yourself. Remember, some word forms add or lose a letter when they are combined with others. Remember, also, that the placement of the hyphens in the word parts shows where they go—at the beginning or end of a word. After you have finished building your words, check a medical dictionary to see how much sense you have made of the language of medicine.

Here are some of the word parts you will find in the section on hematology together with their definitions. Use them to form words that fit the descriptions.

hem- (-o, -a, -ato), blood, Greek

-cyte(o), cell, Greek

erythr-, red, Greek

-poeisis, formation, Greek

-phil(-ia, -ic), love or affinity for, Greek

-meter, instrument for measuring, Greek

-emia, condition of the blood, Greek

bi-, two, Latin

thromb, clot, Greek

neutr(o), neutral, Greek

kary(o), nucleus, Greek

reticul(o), small network, Latin

anti-, counteracting; effective against, Greek

mega-, large, enlargement, Greek

poly-, many, much, Greek

-penia, deficiency, lack, Greek

-sis, condition, Greek

cavum, hollow, Latin

DEFINITIONS THAT NEED A WORD

1. Red cell: _____ .

2. Disease in which there is an abnormal number of white cells in the blood: _____ .

3. Instruments used to measure blood cells: _____ .

4. Process of blood formation: _____ .

5. Cell with a very large nucleus: _____ .

6. Description of a shape that is hollow on both sides: _____ .

7. Blood cell in which a small network shows up after staining: _____ .

8. Condition in which there are fewer than normal neutrophils in the blood: _____ .

9. Condition in which a clot has formed: _____ .

Now that you have tried your hand at building some medical terms, you have probably found that many of them have more than a beginning and an ending. Your instructor will be able to tell you how to decide what order word parts follow in complex terms. Consult the glossary or a medical dictionary if you need help in defining these terms.

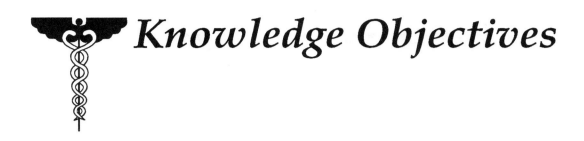

Knowledge Objectives

After completing this chapter, you should be able to:

BLOOD CELLS
- name the major components of the blood
- describe the composition and function of plasma
- describe the origin, composition, and function of erythrocytes
- describe the origin, composition, and function of the two groups of leukocytes
- describe the origin, composition, and function of thrombocytes (platelets)

BLOOD FORMATION, FUNCTION, AND DESTRUCTION
- explain the process of hematopoiesis, and identify the sites at which it takes place
- explain how and where leukocytes are destroyed
- explain how and where erythrocytes are destroyed
- explain coagulation, or the clotting mechanism, and identify the main substances involved in the process
- explain the importance of the acid/base balance of the body, and how the blood maintains it
- explain how blood functions in body temperature regulation

BLOOD GROUPS
- name the major blood groups, and explain the causes of incompatibility
- explain how the Rh factor operates

The Anatomy and Physiology of Blood

INTRODUCTION

Hematology (HEM ah TOL oh jee) is the study of blood. **Blood** is considered a tissue, even though it is fluid. Like lymphatic fluid, it has a fluid **matrix (MAY tricks), (plasma [PLAZ mah])** and also contains cells. Blood has four major functions:

- Transport of oxygen, nutrients, waste products, and other substances within the body
- Defense against foreign substances, including infection
- Regulation of the body's acid/base balance
- Temperature regulation

Blood is not only a red fluid. It has many components. The major ones are plasma—the fluid component—and the blood cells, which are also called the **formed elements**. Plasma is a pale yellow liquid made up of approximately 90 percent water and 10 percent solutes, or substances that dissolve in fluid. These solutes include both solids and gases. Table 1 shows the major solutes found in normal blood plasma. Proteins are the predominant solute in plasma. The others are nutrients, salts, waste products, gases

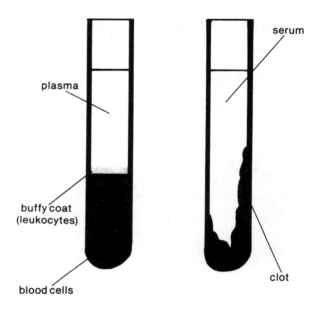

Figure 1: These two test tubes show the differences between blood plasma and blood serum. The dark area in the tube at left represents blood cells centrifuged to the bottom of the tube; leukocytes at the top and erythrocytes below them; the blood plasma is the liquid minus those cells. On the right, the dark area represents a clot—blood cells enmeshed in the fibrin. The liquid remaining after blood has clotted is serum—liquid minus the clotting elements.

(including oxygen), and special protein molecules such as enzymes, hormones, and **antibodies**.

Table 1: Content of the Plasma

Item	Percent	Purpose/Function
Water	91–92%	Liquid medium for transport of blood cells and solutes.
Protein	6–8%	
Albumin		Regulates plasma volume by attracting water from interstitial fluid; binds with nutrients and hormones to keep them in circulation.
Globulins		Transport other proteins and other substances by combining with them; gamma globulins resist infection.
Fibrinogen		Becomes fibrin in clotting process.
Prothrombin		Becomes thrombin in initial stage of clotting process.
Nutrients (Glucose, lipids, amino acids)	Less than 1%	Nourish cells: provide energy and building materials.
Inorganic salts	Less than 1%	Electrolyte balance maintained by circulating sodium chloride.
Gases	Less than 1%	Small amounts of oxygen, carbon dioxide, and nitrogen transported in plasma.
Waste products (Urea, uric acid, lactic acid)	Less than 1%	Transported to intestines and kidneys for elimination.
Hormones	Less than 1%	Transported from endocrine glands to target cells or organs.

Two of the plasma proteins, **prothrombin (proh THROM bin)** and **fibrinogen (fye BRIN oh jen)**, are part of the clotting process. When blood clots (in a test tube, for example), the fluid that remains is called **serum**, not plasma, because these proteins are no longer present and this changes the character of the fluid (see Figure 1).

Another important protein in the plasma is **albumin (al BYOO min)**. It is also the most plentiful of the plasma proteins (55 percent of plasma protein). Albumin is formed in the liver, and its major function is to attract water into the bloodstream from the **interstitial (IN ter STISH al) fluid**. This helps maintain the level of water in the plasma, thus controlling blood volume. Water levels in the plasma are also regulated by the kidneys.

Albumin has a second function as well. It combines with amino acids, fatty acids, hormones, and minerals in the blood, to retain them in the circulation. Most protein molecules are too large to be removed from the blood by the kidneys' filtering units, but amino acids, fatty acids, hormones, and minerals may be filtered out. However, they are needed by the body as nutrients or messengers, so they stick to albumin and remain in the blood.

There are three types of **globulin (GLOB yoo lin)** proteins in plasma: **alpha, beta**, and **gamma**. Like albumin, the globulins can combine with other substances in the plasma, but for a different purpose. Alpha and beta globulins consist of many separate proteins, to carry them to other parts of the body. Gamma globulins, however, are part

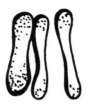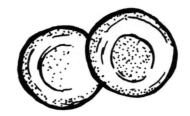

Figure 2: Side (left) and front (right) views of erythrocytes. The side view shows why red blood cells are called biconcave discs. The front view shows the indentation where the nucleus used to be.

of the immune system. They contain antibodies, which resist infection from certain diseases.

The nutrients and oxygen in the plasma are carried to the cells, and replaced by carbon dioxide and other waste products, such as urea and uric acid. The carbon dioxide is returned to the lungs. The urea and uric acid are filtered out of the blood through the kidneys, and excreted in the urine. (See the books on the respiratory system and on urology and the reproductive system, in this series, for details on those functions.)

The plasma also contains blood cells, or **corpuscles (KOR pus ul)**, which means "little bodies." There are three main categories of these cells (see Table 2): **erythrocytes (eh RITH roh syts)**, or red blood cells; **leukocytes (LOO koh syts)**, or white blood cells; and **thrombocytes (THROM boh syts)**, or **platelets (PLAYT lets)**.

ERYTHROCYTES

Erythrocytes, the red blood cells, provide 42 to 47 percent of blood volume. Their job is to transport oxygen from the lungs to the cells, and carbon dioxide back to the lungs. They do this through an important element in their structure, the protein **hemoglobin (HEE moh GLOH bin)**. Hemoglobin has special properties that allow it to combine with and release oxygen and carbon dioxide. It is the oxygen-carrying pigment, which gives erythrocytes their red color.

Erythrocytes are one of the few cell types that do not have nuclei. Immature red blood cells have nuclei, but they are lost in the final stage of red blood cell development. Mature erythrocytes are flexible disks indented in the center both front and back, where the nucleus had been. This form is often referred to as a **biconcave (bye CON kayv) disk**— concave (indented) front and back, so that the center of the disk is thinner than the edges (see Figure 2). Erythrocytes must be flexible so that they can pass through the tiniest arterioles, venules, and capillaries as they circulate. They normally are about the same size, between 6 and 9 microns (abbreviated μ) in diameter with an average diameter of 7.5μ. Variations in size and shape among them are signs of disease.

Red blood cells are formed in the bone marrow. This process is called **erythropoiesis (eh RITH roh poi EE sis)**. Erythrocytes usually survive in the circulation for 105 to 120 days. After this time, they become worn out and do not work effectively. They are destroyed, either by breaking up in the circulation, or by being routed to the spleen or the liver. There, some of the cell components are reclaimed and recycled to the bone marrow, to be used again in making red blood cells. Iron is an essential ingredient in hemoglobin formation, and it is one of the elements that can be recycled in this way.

Another essential ingredient in red blood cell production is **vitamin (VYE tah min)** B_{12}. This vitamin must be obtained from

Table 2: Normal Blood Cell Characteristics

Cell Type	Description	Average Number	Function	Formation/ Destruction
Erythrocyte (red blood cell)	7μ diameter, biconcave disk, no nucleus.	Males: 5.5 mill. per cu. mm. Females: 4.8 mill. per cu. mm.	Transport oxygen from lungs to cells and carbon dioxide from cells to lungs.	Formed in red bone marrow. Destroyed after 105–120 days, in capillaries, spleen, liver, and red bone marrow.
Leukocytes (white blood cells)	(See specific types.)	5,000–9,000 per cu. mm.	Immunity	Lifespan not known. Thought to be 3–12 days, except for some small lymphocytes.
Thrombocytes (platelets)	2–4μ dia. Colorless, oval or irregular discs.	Average of 250,000/cu. mm.	Stop blood flow from injured vessels, part of clotting mechanism.	Formed in red bone marrow, lungs, spleen. Lifespan about 10 days. Destruction mechanism unknown.
Reticulocyte	Immature rbc, has granules remaining from nucleus	0.5–1.5% of rbc's	Same as rbc's, when mature.	Formed in red bone marrow. Become mature cells, same cycle as rbc's.
Granular leukocytes				
Neutrophil (polymorphonuclear leuk., or "polys")	10–15μ dia. Nucleus with 4–5 lobes. Granules stain pink to violet in Wright's stain.	# varies—increases in infection. Normally 65% of wbc's.	Phagocytosis of microbes and other foreign material.	Formed in red bone marrow. Destroyed sometimes by bacteria, sometimes by unknown causes.
Eosinophil	10–15μ dia. Granules stain orange in acid dye (eosin), red in Wright's stain. Nucleus has 2 lobes.	Average is 3% of wbc	May detoxify blood of proteins in allergic reactions.	Formed in red bone marrow. Destruction mechanism unknown.
Basophil	10–15μ dia. S-shaped nucleus. Large granules stain purple in basic dye, bluish-black in Wright's stain.	Average is 1% of wbc's	Function unclear; may prevent abnormal clotting.	Formed in red bone marrow. Destruction mechanism unknown.
Nongranular leukocytes				
Lymphocytes (B-cells and T-cells)	Large nucleus, small cytoplasm. Largest 8μ dia., also in smaller size.	Average is 25% of wbc's	Form antibodies against foreign substances, including viruses.	Formed in lymph tissue—nodes and spleen. Also in red bone marrow. Some small cells may survive 100–200 days.
Monocytes	15–20μ dia. Kidney-shaped nucleus.	Average 6% of wbc's	Phagocytosis of bacteria and other invaders.	Formed in lymph tissue—nodes and spleen. Also in red bone marrow.

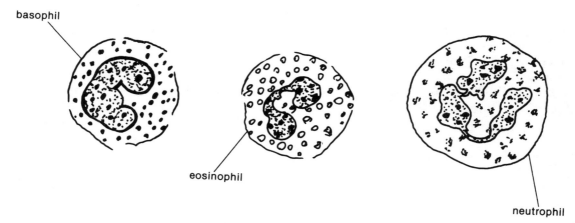

basophil

eosinophil

neutrophil

Figure 3: The three types of granular leukocytes

food. It enters the stomach, is absorbed into the bloodstream, and is delivered to the liver for storage. In order for B_{12} to be absorbed, cells in the stomach lining must produce a substance called **intrinsic (in TRIN sick) factor**. Without this substance, the body cannot use B_{12}; it passes through the digestive system without being absorbed. Once it has been absorbed and stored, the vitamin is available and is released by the liver to the bone marrow as needed. Other essential ingredients in red cell production are copper, cobalt, folic acid, pyridoxine, and protein.

Production of red cells goes on continuously as older cells wear out and are destroyed, and new cells are needed to replace them. These cells go through several stages of maturation, ending as mature erythrocytes. They then enter the bloodstream. The stage just before maturity is called the **reticulocyte (reh TICK yoo loh syt)**. Normally, 0.5 to 1.5 percent of red cells in the circulation are reticulocytes, which have lost their nuclei but still retain a few granules of ribosomes in the **cytoplasm (SYE toh plazm)** or the interior of the cell. When there is a shortage of red blood cells in the circulation, the proportion of reticulo-

cytes increases as the mechanism of erythropoiesis speeds up.

LEUKOCYTES

Leukocytes are also known as white blood cells or white corpuscles. There are fewer of them than of erythrocytes in the blood, but they are larger and there are five different types instead of one. Leukocytes fall into two groups: **granular (GRAN yoo lar)** and **nongranular (non GRAN yoo lar)**. These groups differ in the appearance of the cytoplasm. Three of the five types, the granular leukocytes, have granules in the cytoplasm that show up under a microscope when different stains are applied to a blood smear on a slide (see Figure 3). The other two types, the nongranular leukocytes, do not have these granules. Each of the five types has its own specific function, although not all of these functions are completely understood. In general, leukocytes are the "clean-up squad" of the body, and function as part of the immune system. As they circulate, they can leave the blood vessels and enter the interstitial fluid. Once there, they engulf and digest foreign material such as bacteria and fragments of broken cells. This process is called **phagocytosis (FAG oh sye TOH sis)**.

Granular Leukocytes

The three granular leukocytes are **neutrophils (NYOO troh filz)**, **eosinophils (EE oh SIN oh filz)**, and **basophils (BAY soh filz)** (see Figure 3 and Table 2). These names come from the Greek root *phil* (FIL), which means to love, combined with the Latin term for *neutral*, and Greek term for a type of acid and base. The granules in the cells attract (love) dyes with different pH ratings. You can tell the cells apart by staining a blood smear with neutral, acid, and basic dyes, and observing the color of the granules and the nucleus. A stain called Wright's stain, which is a combination of acid and basic dyes, is often used to stain blood smears.

The shape of the nucleus also varies by the cell type. Neutrophils are the most numerous, not just of the granular leukocytes, but of all the white blood cells. They are from 10 to 15µ in diameter. The nuclei of these cells have between two and five lobules, and stain a purplish-blue with Wright's stain. The granules are small and stain pink to violet. Neutrophils are also called **polymorphonuclear (POL ee MOR foh NYOO clee ar) leukocytes**, meaning that they have many-shaped nuclei. This is sometimes shortened to **polys (POL eez)**.

Neutrophils also are the most mobile of the white blood cells. In bacterial infections, the number of neutrophils increases to fight the disease. During an infection, immature forms of neutrophils, called **band cells**, may appear in the circulation, as the bone marrow hurries to increase the supply. These cells have horseshoe-shaped nuclei.

Eosinophils make up only 1 to 3 percent of the leukocytes. They have nuclei with two, or sometimes three, oval lobules, and their large, numerous granules stain orange with acid dyes (eosins) or red with Wright's stain. The cells are 10 to 15µ in diameter. In allergic reactions and parasitic infections, the number of eosinophils in the blood increases. It is thought that these cells detoxify foreign proteins in the body, but this is not fully established. These cells move far more slowly than the neutrophils.

Basophils are smaller than neutrophils and eosinophils, being only 8 to 14µ in diameter. The nucleus of a basophil is covered with a few large granules so that its S shape is hard to see. The granules stain dark purple with basic dyes, or bluish-black with Wright's stain.

Basophils make up less than 1 percent of the leukocytes. Their function is not known, but they do contain an **anticoagulant (AN tih koh AG yoo lant)**, **heparin (HEP ah rin)**, which may have something to do with their function.

Nongranular Leukocytes

The two types of nongranular leukocytes are **lymphocytes (LIM foh syts)** and **monocytes (MON oh syts)** (Figure 4 and Table 2). Lymphocytes exist in two sizes, large and small. The average size is 8µ in diameter—smaller than most granular leukocytes, but slightly larger than an erythrocyte. The nucleus in a lymphocyte is large and round, with a notch or indentation in one side. A thin layer of cytoplasm surrounds the nucleus. These cells make up 20 to 25 percent of the white blood cells.

Lymphocytes come in three forms: undifferentiated, and differentiated into either **B-cells** or **T-cells**. B-cells form antibodies that attack antigens, or foreign proteins. Some T-cells are named for the **thymus**

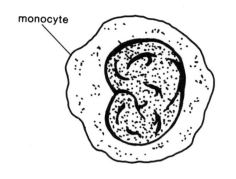
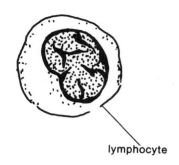

monocyte

lymphocyte

Figure 4: Nongranular leukocytes

(THYE mus), a small organ located in the chest and throat that is part of the lymphatic system, because undifferentiated lymphocytes are changed to T-cells in the thymus. In the acquired immunodeficiency syndrome (AIDS), the human immunodeficiency virus attacks these T-cells. The cells are then unable to fight infection. When the blood level of lymphocytes falls below 200 per mm^3 the risk of a serious AIDS-defining infection is very likely. (AIDS is discussed in greater detail later in this book.)

Monocytes (see Figure 4) are the largest of the leukocytes, with diameters of 15 to 20μ. They make up 3 to 8 percent of the white blood cells. The nucleus of a monocyte is kidney-shaped, and small in relation to the cell as a whole. The cytoplasm is grayish.

Monocytes operate in much the same way as neutrophils. They travel to a site of damage or infection, and phagocytose (digest) foreign material. Monocytes specialize in removing larger particles, such as parts of damaged cells, while neutrophils deal mainly with bacteria.

THROMBOCYTES (PLATELETS)

The final type of formed element in the blood is the thrombocyte, or platelet (see Table 4). Thrombocytes are smaller than other blood cells, only 2 to 5μ in diameter.

They are irregular in shape, and have granules but no nuclei (see Figure 5). Thrombocytes are not really cells, but fragments of larger cells called **megakaryocytes (MEG ah KAR ee oh syts)** that remain in the bone marrow.

The function of thrombocytes is to help prevent blood loss. When a small tear occurs in a blood vessel, thrombocytes adhere to the damaged area and form a plug to fill the hole and prevent blood from leaking into the surrounding tissues. If the damage is more extensive, a **blood clot** is also needed, and the thrombocytes have an important role in clot formation, or **coagulation (koh AG yoo LAY shun)**. Coagulation can also occur in the bloodstream in the absence of an injury. It can be caused by deposits or roughening in the vessel walls, prolonged inactivity (as in a bedridden patient), and other conditions that interfere with normal blood flow (see Figure 6). Some experts believe that blood constantly coagulates and dissolves as it flows though the veins and arteries.

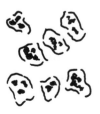

Figure 5: Thrombocytes

Fill in the blanks

1. The major components of blood are _____ (the
    _____ component), and _____ .

2. Plasma is made up of about _____% water and _____% solutes.

3. Solutes in plasma include proteins, such as _____ and
    _____, which are part of the clotting process.

4. The major function of albumin is to attract _____into the blood
    from the _____ fluid.

5. One of the globulin proteins in plasma is part of the immune system; it is called
    _____ globulin.

6. The three main types blood cells are _____, _____, and _____ .

True or False

7. Erythrocytes transport carbon dioxide from the lungs to the cells, and carry oxygen
    back to the lungs. T/F

8. Erythrocytes are a type of body cell that never have nuclei. T/F

9. Leukocytes are able to leave the blood vessels and enter the interstitial fluid. T/F

10. B-cells are changed to T-cells by the thymus. T/F

Fill in the blanks

11. Mature erythrocytes must be flexible in shape because they must _____
    _____ .

12. Erythrocytes that are not shaped like biconcave discs are signs of _____
    _____ .

13. Erythrocytes are formed in the _____ marrow.

14. Vitamin _____ is an essential component in red blood cells.

15. The presence of more than 1.5% of reticulocytes in the circulation indicates that
    _____ .

16. White blood cells are called _____ .

17. Leukocytes whose names end in -phil attract different _____ ;
    because of this, staining a blood smear with _____, which
    is a combination of acid and basic dyes, can be used to identify these different types
    of white blood cells.

(continued next page)

18. The nuclei of _____, the most numerous of all the white blood cells, appear purplish-blue with small pink to violet granules when they are stained with _____ .

19. The percentage of eosinophils in the blood increases during _____ .

20. Nongranular leukocytes are of two types: _____, and _____.

21. The three forms of lymphocytes are _____, _____, and _____ .

22. The lymphocyte that forms antibodies is the _____ .

23. Monocytes, the second type of leukocyte, are activated by _____ .

24. Monocytes function similarly to neutrophils; both move to a site of damage or infection to _____ .

25. The main function of thrombocytes is to form _____ to help prevent _____ from damaged blood vessels.

BLOOD FORMATION, FUNCTION, AND DESTRUCTION

Hematopoiesis

The term **hematopoiesis (HEM ah toh poi EE sis)** means formation of blood cells. The process of cell formation is crucial, because blood cells constantly wear out or are destroyed, and they must be replaced constantly to maintain the proper amounts of formed elements in the blood.

Most blood cells are made in the red bone marrow, which is the most cellular part of the bone marrow. The only exceptions are lymphocytes and monocytes, most of which are made in the lymphatic system, although some are made in bone marrow. In certain disease states, thrombocytes as well as red cells and neutrophils can be made in other parts of the body—the spleen, lung, and liver.

All these formed elements probably derive from a common parent, the **primordial (prye MOR dee al)**, or **hematopoietic (HEM ah toh poi ET ick) stem cell**. These primitive cells remain in the bone marrow (and also in the lymphatic system and other organs) and replicate (reproduce) constantly by dividing through a process called **mitosis (mye TOH sis)**. Mitosis produces cells called **daughter cells**, which differentiate into primitive forms of the various blood cells. These primitive cells gradually mature. They pass through several stages of growth and development before they are finally released into the bloodstream.

Early stages are designated by the suffix -blast, and later stages by the suffix -cyte, meaning cell. For example, an **erythroblast (eh RITH roh blast)** is a primitive erythrocyte, and a **lymphoblast (LIM foh blast)** is an early form of a lymphocyte. Usually the immature forms of these cells remain in the bone marrow, but, as we have seen, normal blood may contain some reticulocytes (immature red blood cells) and band cells (immature neutrophils). The immature cells can be seen in examination of the bone marrow, as well as in the blood in certain blood diseases or severe infections in which the manufacture of cells cannot keep up with their destruction.

Different blood cells have different normal lifespans, depending on their function. Red blood cells normally live for 105 to 120 days; thrombocytes live only about 10 days. Most white blood cells have a short lifespan since their purpose is to engage in warfare with invaders. Naturally there are casualties. When neutrophils and other white blood cells are overwhelmed by an infection, disease occurs.

The residue of defeated white blood cells, mixed with bacteria, active cells, and dead tissue cells, forms the material known as **pus**. Pus signifies at least a temporary defeat of the immune system by bacterial invasion. Similarly, when a patient with a respiratory infection coughs up mucus mixed with yellowish or greenish pus, this often indicates a bacterial infection rather than a viral infection; that is, bronchitis rather than a mere cold. Bronchitis is potentially a more serious illness, but it can be treated with antibiotics, which will not help defeat a viral infection.

It is not known how white blood cells are destroyed, or exactly how long they live. Probably most live from 3 to 12 days, but a few lymphocytes have been found to live up to 200 days, and possibly even longer.

The destruction of red blood cells is understood much better. The linings of the blood vessels, the liver, the spleen, and the bone marrow are equipped with **reticuloendothelial (reh TICK yoo loh EN do THEE lee al) cells**. These cells, which are part of the immune system, remain stationary. As worn-out, broken, or abnormal red blood cells come into contact with them, the reticuloendothelial cells digest or phagocytose them. This normally occurs at a rate of about 100 million cells per minute. Red blood cells normally are replaced at the same rate.

The life cycle of thrombocytes, which are not complete cells but only cell fragments, is somewhat different. Thrombocytes break off from large (49 to 170μ in diameter) megakaryocytes, cells that form from primitive stem cells in the marrow, spleen, and lungs, but remain in those locations. As thrombocytes are needed, they break off from the cytoplasm of these larger cells and enter the circulation. When the thrombocytes are needed to seal up a blood vessel or form a clot, they adhere to the blood vessel wall and disintegrate, releasing chemicals required for coagulation (see Figure 6). Thus, thrombocytes necessarily are destroyed as they perform their normal function.

Coagulation

The coagulation or **clotting mechanism** is a complex chemical process. (The explanation given here is simplified.) When a wound occurs, thrombocytes adhere to the rough place, tear, or a deposit in a blood vessel wall. The thrombocytes release chemicals (called **platelet factors**) that accelerate the coagulation reaction and constrict the surrounding blood vessels. Prothrombin in the plasma reacts with platelet factors and calcium and changes to thrombin.

Thrombin then reacts with fibrinogen in the plasma, causing the fibrinogen to uncoil into long threads called **fibrin (FYE brin)**. Fibrin forms a net that traps red blood cells and holds the thrombocytes in place at the site of the original injury or abnormality, forming a clot (see Figure 6). Eventually, an enzyme present in the blood called **fibrinolysin (FYE brih NOL ih sin)** dissolves the

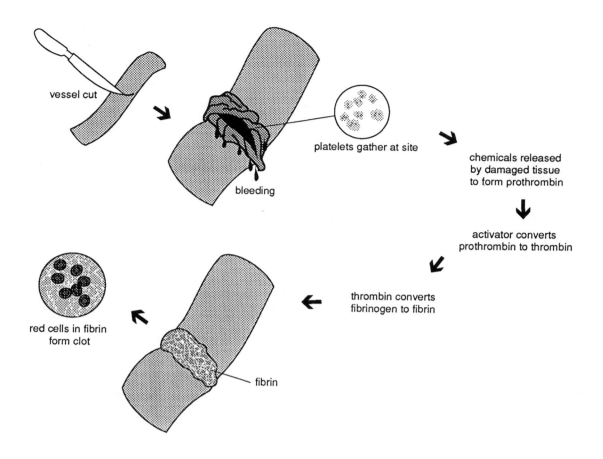

vessel cut

bleeding

platelets gather at site

chemicals released
by damaged tissue
to form prothrombin

activator converts
prothrombin to thrombin

thrombin converts
fibrinogen to fibrin

red cells in fibrin
form clot

fibrin

Figure 6: Coagulation

fibrin, and the clot disappears.

The process of coagulation and **fibrinolysis (FYE brih NOL ih sis)** called **lysis (LYE sis)**, or the destruction of fibrin, goes on continuously as small injuries occur in the capillaries. A balance must be maintained between excessive clotting and insufficient clotting, to ensure continuous blood flow through the circulatory system. Substances called **antithrombins (AN tih THROM binz)**, which oppose the action of thrombin in the clotting process, circulate in the blood. One of these is heparin, which is found in basophils and also is used as an anticoagulant in blood specimens.

Another essential factor in maintaining the clotting process is vitamin K. This substance must be present in the liver before prothrombin can be made. Vitamin K is found in some foods (such as spinach and other leafy, green vegetables) and also is made by special bacteria in the intestines. Newborn babies often have a deficiency of this vitamin, and therefore a prothrombin deficiency. For this reason, supplemental vitamin K is given to most newborns.

Acid/Base Balance

The blood has another function that is related to its chemical content rather than to the formed elements. It is the center of the mechanisms that maintain the proper **acid/base balance**, or **pH**. The blood normally has a very narrow range of pH, between 7.35 and 7.45, or slightly alkaline (base). (For a review of pH, see the book on bio-organization in this series.)

It is crucial for body fluids to remain within this range, with two major exceptions. These are the stomach fluids and the urine. In the stomach, hydrochloric acid is a major component of the digestive juices. Therefore, the stomach is much more acidic than any other area of the body. The urine is a major fluid by which the body eliminates excess acid, so it too is more acidic than other body fluids, and this affects the pH of the kidneys and the rest of the urinary tract.

Elsewhere in the body, the slightly alkaline environment of the plasma is necessary so that cells can function properly. Most hormones and enzymes, the body's messengers and facilitators, require a pH within the range described to work effectively. As we have seen, the plasma, lymph, and interstitial fluid are all very similar in chemical composition, and these fluids also are in constant flux. Plasma enters the spaces between the cells with its supply of nutrients and oxygen, blends with the interstitial fluid, and is drained back into the blood vessels and the lymphatic system.

Three major mechanisms maintain the acid/base balance in the blood and thus in body fluids in general. These mechanisms are the respiratory system, the kidneys, and chemical **buffers** in the blood.

Acid and basic substances enter the body through the digestive system, and are broken down and absorbed. The cells make carbon dioxide as they use oxygen, and carbon dioxide forms carbonic acid in the blood. The balance mechanisms counteract these inputs into the system.

When excess acid is detected in the blood by internal sensors, the respiratory system and urinary system eliminate it. Breathing speeds up to eliminate more carbon dioxide and add more oxygen. At the same time, the kidneys increase the amount of acid they are filtering out of the blood. If the blood becomes too alkaline, breathing slows down and the kidneys retain more acid instead of eliminating it. These measures are not needed except in extreme changes in the acid/base balance. Usually such situations are prevented by the buffering mechanism.

The plasma solutes include weak acids and weak bases that combine with stronger acids or bases as they enter the blood. The effect is to dilute the acidity or alkalinity of these elements, and so keep changes in pH to a minimum.

If all three mechanisms fail, either **acidosis (AS ih DOH sis)** or **alkalosis (AL kah LOH sis)** occurs. In untreated acidosis, the patient becomes drowsy, then comatose, and eventually dies. In alkalosis, excessive neuromuscular excitability, confusion, seizures, and **arrhythmias (ah RITH mee ahz)** may occur.

Temperature Regulation

The blood also serves as part of the regulatory mechanism of internal body temperature. The **hypothalamus (HYE poh THAL ah mus)**, which is part of the brain, monitors the temperature of the blood. When the temperature rises above a certain level, usually 37°C, two things happen: the sweat glands are stimulated to produce more sweat, and the blood vessels near the surface of the skin dilate, or open. The blood carries heat to the skin's surface, where the sweat evaporates, thus cooling the surface. When the body's thermostat registers that the temperature is too low, the surface blood vessels constrict, or close. The warmth in the blood stays away from the skin's surface, and is retained by the body. At the same time, the body involuntarily shivers, causing muscle activity that in turn generates body heat. In either case, the blood transports body heat to the appropriate area. Then it can be dissipated or conserved, whichever is needed.

Inflammatory Response

When cells are damaged, by microbes, physical causes, or chemical agents, a complex series of events follows that involves the chemicals and cells we have been discussing. No matter what the cause, the **inflammatory (in FLAM ah TOH ree) response** is often the same. The injury is seen by the body as a form of stress, and the body's nonspecific internal defense systems go into action immediately. Chemical mediators, mostly enzymes and hormones, are released in response to tissue damage. These mediators, including **histamine (HIS tah meen), prostaglandins (PROS tah GLAN dinz), complement (KOM pleh ment)** and **kinins (KIH ninz)** cause the vessels to dilate, increasing the blood flow, and bringing phagocytes and leukocytes to the area. They also increase vascular permeability, allowing fibrin, complement, and kinins to enter the tissues. Complement and kinins in the tissue accelerate the inflammatory process. The process of increasing the numbers of chemical mediators and attracting phagocytes continues until the bacteria are destroyed. If the causative bacteria are destroyed, the white blood cells clean the site of infection.

Pus is present in all but the very mildest of inflammations. It continues to be present to some degree until the infection has cleared. If pus cannot drain from the body, an **abscess (AB ses)** develops. An abscess is the accumulation of pus in a confined space. Since an abscess cannot drain, it must be surgically opened and the pus allowed to escape. Boils are a common form of abscess.

It is the increased blood flow and vascular permeability that produce the symptoms of redness, heat, and swelling at the site of infection. Swelling, as well as the chemical mediators acting on the nerve cells, produces pain. The temporary loss of function comes from the swelling too, and also from pain and tissue damage itself.

A local inflammation is confined to a specific area of the body. However, the inflammatory response can also occur on a systemic level. In a systemic inflammation, such as a viral infection, the inflammatory response occurs in many parts of the body at the same time. In addition to the symptoms of local inflammation, caused by cellular damage, there is also fever. This is due to the fever-producing agents called pyrogens, which are released by microorganisms, **macrophages (MACK roh fahjz)**, neutrophils, and other cells. Fever stimulates the activity of the immune system.

BLOOD GROUPS

The first blood **transfusions (trans FYOO zhunz)** were attempted by several scientists, in the 17th century, with disappointing results. Blood from humans and animals was used. A few patients recovered, but others did not. In 1900, Karl Landsteiner discovered blood types or groups, and clarified why the original experiments were not wholly successful. Today it is commonly understood that one person's blood cannot be mixed indiscriminately with someone else's. This is due to the presence of two factors in the blood: **markers** or **antigens (AN tih jen)**, also called **agglutinogens (AG loo TIN oh jenz)**, on the red blood cells and antibodies in the plasma.

If an incompatible blood type is used in a transfusion, the antibodies in the recipient's blood will cause the foreign red blood cells to **agglutinate (ah GLOO tih nayt)**, or clump together. An individual's blood falls within one of four major groups or types according to the combination of antigens

STOP AND REVIEW

True or False

1. Blood cells are made in the red bone marrow, except for neutrophils and monocytes.

Circle one

2. A lymphoblast appears as an earlier/later form than a lymphocyte.

Fill in the blanks

3. The parent, or _____ cell from which all _____ or blood cells derive, is found in the _____, where it reproduces by mitosis.

4. An immature neutrophil is called a(n) _____.

5. Pus is composed of _____.

6. The formed element in the blood that is actually part of a larger cell is the _____ _____.

7. The process of coagulation involves thrombocytes, which release _____ that speed up coagulation reaction, _____ that reacts with those chemicals and calcium to produce thrombin, and fibrinogen, that reacts with _____ to produce fibrin, which together with red blood cells and thrombocytes, forms a _____.

8. A substance that prevents excessive clotting is _____, found in basophils. This substance is used as an anticoagulant in blood specimens.

9. Most body fluids must remain within a slightly alkaline pH range. The exceptions are the _____ and the _____.

10. If the blood is excessively acid, the _____ and _____ increase their activity to eliminate _____ and add oxygen.

11. The part of the brain that monitors blood temperature is the _____.

Table 3: Antigens and Antibodies in the Major Blood Groups

Group	Antigens on Red Blood Cells	Antibodies in Plasma
A	A	Anti-B
B	B	Anti-A
AB	A and B	none
O	none	Anti-A and Anti-B

and antibodies. The **blood groups** are known as A, B, AB, and 0 (see Table 3).

This unique system protects each individual against the blood of other groups. A person with type A blood is protected against type B blood by the presence of B antibodies in the plasma. A person with type B blood is protected against type A cells by anti-A antibodies in the plasma (see Figure 7). Those with the A and B antigen on their red cells have no antibodies against A or B antigens, and those who have type O blood have both kinds of antibodies, anti-A and anti-B.

The problem in **transfusion reactions** is the clumping of donated red blood cells called **agglutination (ah GLOO tih NAY shun)** caused by the antibodies in the recipient's blood (see Figure 8). Therefore type O is considered **universal donor** blood type—it has no "aggravating" antigens on the red cells. Type AB is considered the **universal recipient** type, because it has no antibodies in the plasma that will cause agglutination when combined with antigens on any red blood cells. However, factors other than A and B antigens and antibodies can cause transfusion reactions, even when so-called universal donor or universal recipient blood is involved.

If red blood cells contain a protein called the **Rh factor**, the individual's blood is said to be **Rh-positive**; if the blood cells do not contain this antigen, the person's blood is **Rh-negative**. This additional factor was discovered by Landsteiner and a colleague in 1937, based on experiments with rhesus monkeys. Approximately 15 percent of populations of Western European descent have Rh-negative blood. All the others have Rh-positive blood. The distribution is different for other racial groups. The Rh type is also referred to as a "D antigen" or "0 type."

The presence of ABO and Rh antigens can be determined by using **antisera (AN tih SEE rah) (singular: antiserum [AN tih SEE rum])**. An antiserum is a commercially prepared pure suspension of antibodies that will react only with a specific antigen. For example, the blood of a person with A antigen on the surface of the red cells will agglutinate when mixed with anti-A antiserum, and so on. The antisera can be added to drops of a blood specimen on a slide, to determine the blood type of the specimen.

Before a transfusion can be done safely, donated blood must be cross-matched directly with the patient's blood in a similar procedure. Even if the donated blood is the same type, differing subgroups can still cause agglutination in the body. This in turn prevents the blood from circulating normally, and can cause severe illness and even death. Even when all known precautions are taken, transfusions are not always safe and effective. Adverse reactions, called transfusion reactions, are not 100 percent predictable outside the body.

The Rh factor is important in pregnancy, should the mother have Rh-negative blood and the father have Rh-positive blood. In such a case, the fetus may have Rh-positive blood, since blood types are inherited. With the first child, this usually causes no problems, since maternal and fetal blood normally do not mix. However, in late pregnancy or during delivery, there is usually some mixing of the blood. The mother's immune system then builds up antibodies against the Rh factor. This can also occur in a miscarriage or an abortion. If a later pregnancy produces another Rh-positive fetus, the mother's blood will contain antibodies that attack the fetal red blood cells.

Although the mother's red blood cells do not cross the placenta into the fetal blood, the antibodies are much smaller and can cross that barrier. The result is agglutination of the fetal blood cells, a disease called **erythroblastosis fetalis (eh RITH roh blas TOH sis feh TAY lis)**. If it is not treated, this condition can damage or kill the fetus. A substance called **RhoGAM** is available that prevents formation of antibodies against the Rh factor. It is a concentrated gamma globu-

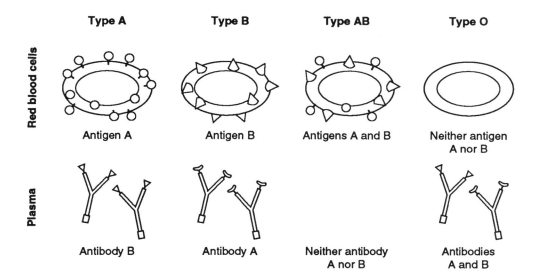

Figure 7: ABO blood groups

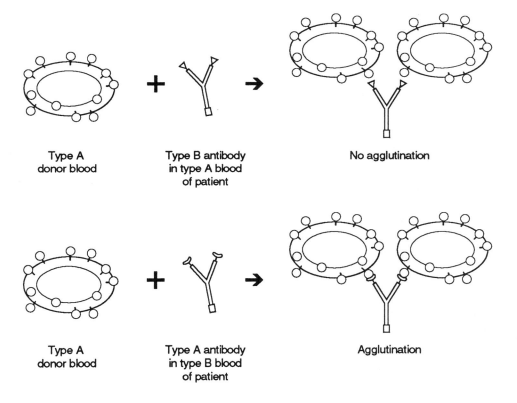

Figure 8: Agglutination reactions

Table 4: Distribution of ABO Blood Types in Three United States Groups

Type	Caucasian	African	Asian
A	45%	29%	35%
B	8%	17%	23%
AB	4%	4%	12%
O	43%	50%	30%

Source: William J. Williams, et. al. Hematology (3rd Edition) McGraw-Hill, NY, 1983, p. 1494.

lin that is active specifically against the Rh antigen. It is obtained from the serum of women who have had a baby affected with erythroblastosis. RhoGAM destroys any fetal blood cells in the mother's blood before antibodies to those cells can form. Since most fetal blood cells enter the mother's circulation when the baby is born, giving RhoGAM at birth is effective in avoiding Rh-factor problems in later pregnancies.

As Table 4 shows, blood types are distributed differently among different racial groups. Like race, blood type is inherited. According to some experts, every person's blood is as unique as his or her fingerprints.

STOP AND REVIEW

Fill in the blanks

1. One person's blood cannot be indiscriminately mixed with another person's blood because of _____ on the red blood cells and _____ in the plasma.

Matching

2. Mix and match blood group, antigen, and antibody.

GROUP	ANTIGEN	ANTIBODY
A_____	None	Anti-A & Anti-B
B_____	A & B	None
AB_____	A	Anti-B
O_____	B	Anti-A

True or False

3. Blood types are differently distributed among different racial groups. T/F

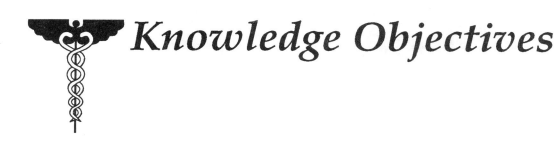

Knowledge Objectives

After completing this chapter, you should be able to:

- list the types of abnormalities of formed elements that may be present in blood diseases
- name the two major approaches to treatment of blood disorders
- list the three major groups of blood tests and give some examples of each
- describe five erythrocyte abnormalities
- describe the causes and treatment of some forms of anemia
- describe the causes and treatment of some inherited blood diseases
- describe the causes and treatment of some neoplastic blood diseases
- describe the causes and treatment of septicemia

Blood Diseases

INTRODUCTION

Most blood diseases involve abnormalities in the formed elements of the blood, the blood cells. The abnormalities may be in the number of cells (too many or too few, their shape, how they are made, or their composition. **Anemia (ah NEE mee ah)** is the best known of the blood disorders, and also the most common. In anemia the body has an inadequate supply of erythrocytes (red blood cells), or not enough hemoglobin in those cells, or both. Anemia has many possible causes, and can be a symptom of diseases that are not directly related to the blood.

We have seen that abnormal blood characteristics are inherited. Some of the best known of these are **sickle (SICK ul) cell anemia**, an abnormality of the red blood cells, and **hemophilia (HEE moh FIL ee ah)**, an abnormality of the clotting mechanism.

Another well-known blood disease is **leukemia (loo KEE mee ah)**, which is a malignancy of the white blood cells. There are several forms of leukemia, and some are more severe and more difficult to treat than others.

The most valuable tools in diagnosis of blood disorders are found in the hematology laboratory. Blood tests are also extremely important in diagnosis of other diseases, because the blood travels throughout the body and therefore often reflects imbalances and abnormalities of other systems. A good example is the elevation of the **white blood cell count** in the circulation, particularly neutrophils, that is seen when an infection is present somewhere in the body. Also, the chemical content of the plasma (or serum) changes in known ways in the presence of certain diseases, such as liver diseases and after a heart attack.

There are two major approaches to treatment of blood disorders: drugs and nutritional supplements to restore balance, and the transfusion, or replacement, of lost or damaged blood. Another approach is **bone marrow transplantation (MAR oh TRANS plan TAY shun)**. Since blood cells are made in the marrow, certain disorders of cell manufacture can be treated by replacing diseased marrow with donated marrow. The donated tissue must be carefully matched to that of the recipient, or the transplant will be rejected by the immune system.

DIAGNOSIS OF BLOOD DISORDERS

Blood tests fall into three major groups: direct examination of the blood, including blood cell counts; chemical tests; and **coagulation tests**. For the first two types and some coagulation tests, blood must be taken from the patient. This can be done by the fingerstick method, in which only a few drops are taken by piercing a finger (or an earlobe or a heel) with a lancet. It can be done by venipuncture, in which a needle is inserted into a certain vein to remove a larger quantity of blood. Depending on what tests are needed, drawn blood may require certain additives, such as anticoagulants to prevent clotting, or preservatives if the blood is to be sent to a laboratory for testing or if tests will be delayed. Blood specimens are fragile and must be handled gently to prevent coagulation or damage to the formed elements. For some tests the blood is centrifuged, or spun at a high speed, to cause the formed elements to fall to the bottom of the test tube. The liquid (either serum or plasma) can then be poured off and tested. Serum is acquired by allowing the blood to clot before pouring off the remaining fluid.

EXAMINATION OF WHOLE BLOOD

This group of tests is done to observe the formed elements of the blood (see Table 2). Some common tests are defined below, and the procedures described very briefly. Detailed instructions about performing these tests can be found in the book on laboratory processes in this series.

Hemoglobin
A hemoglobin test, which can be done by one of several instruments, measures the amount of the molecule hemoglobin present in a blood sample.

Hematocrit
A **hematocrit (hee MAT oh krit)** is a measurement of the percentage of total blood volume occupied by red blood cells. One method that is commonly used is the **microhematocrit** method. A small amount of

whole blood is poured into a small test tube and centrifuged. When the red cells are separated out of the blood, a scale (provided with the equipment) measures the proportion of red cells. Another method for determining the hematocrit is the Wintrobe or **macrohematocrit method,** which requires the use of a larger (Wintobe) tube and more blood. The results indicate the presence of anemia.

Erythrocyte Sedimentation Rate (ESR)
Blood with an anticoagulant added is poured into a thin tube. The rate at which the red blood cells settle in the tube (the sedimentation rate) is measured after the tube has been hung in the vertical position for 1 hour. The ESR increases in inflammatory diseases such as arthritis and rheumatic fever. It detects the presence of inflammation, but does not indicate the source or the cause of the inflammation. The ESR provides a way to help the physician determine whether treatment is effective.

White Blood Cell Count
A blood sample is diluted with a fluid that also **lyses (LYZ es),** or destroys, the mature red blood cells. Any immature red cells, as well as leukocytes and platelets, remain intact. The fluid is then poured into a tiny device called a **hemacytometer (HEM ah sye TOM eh ter),** or counting chamber; the cells are then counted under the microscope. The cells can also be counted by a machine made for that purpose.

Platelet Count
Platelets can be counted in the same way as white blood cells, but since they are smaller the magnification is increased.

Red Blood Cell Count
In this procedure, a different **diluent (DIL yoo ent)** is added to the blood specimen to

preserve the erythrocytes rather than lysing them. The process is similar to the one for counting white blood cells. Again, the procedure can be done automatically instead of manually if the proper equipment is available.

Differential Blood Cell Count

This test is done to estimate how many of each type of white cell are present, and to determine whether all the cells are normal and mature. A blood specimen is carefully smeared onto a slide, so that the cells are spread out evenly but not damaged. The slide is then stained, often with a preparation called Wright's stain, which contains acid and basic dyes. The stain reveals the differences between the various types of white blood cells. When the specimen has dried, the slide is examined under a microscope. The white cells are counted, and all the cells (including erythrocytes) are observed for shape, color, and other characteristics.

Reticulocyte Count

A few drops of whole anticoagulated blood are added to a test tube with a blue stain designed to highlight RNA (a remnant of the nucleus) in red blood cells. Slides are made from this mixture, and examined under a microscope. The normal red cells and the reticulocytes, or immature red cells, are counted on at least two slides, up to 500 cells on each slide. The percentage of reticulocytes is then compared to the percentage of red cells. This test indicates whether the bone marrow is producing red cells at a normal rate. Excessive numbers of reticulocytes indicate that the marrow is attempting to make up for a red cell deficit.

Examination of Red Blood Cells

A slide of a specimen of whole blood is made and stained, usually with Wright's stain. It is then examined under a microscope to determine whether the red blood cells are normal. Some terms describing abnormalities of erythrocytes are listed in Table 5.

BLOOD CHEMISTRY TESTS

The level of a specific chemical in the blood can be determined by clinical chemistry tests. A common method is **spectrophotometry (SPECK troh foh TOM eh tree)**. One or more reagents are added to a specimen of whole blood plasma or serum (usually serum) to stimulate or dilute a color in the specimen. The intensity of this color is measured in a device called a **spectrophotometer (SPECK troh foh TOM eh ter)**, and the result is compared to normal measures.

Clinical chemistry tests measure hemoglobin (in whole blood), protein, glucose, uric acid, cholesterol, specific enzymes, and many other substances. Most of these tests are not used to diagnose blood disorders as such, but to help diagnose other disorders that are reflected in changes in blood chemistry. An important exception is the hemoglobin measurement. This test can be done in conjunction with a hematocrit test (which measures the relative volume of red blood cells) to diagnose anemia.

COAGULATION TESTS

Many tests can be done to measure various aspects of the clotting ability of a patient's blood. In the **bleeding time test**, a small incision is made in the patient's skin and the time required for bleeding to stop is recorded. The result is compared to a known standard.

Another test is called the **prothrombin time test**. A blood specimen is taken from the patient and an anticoagulant that pre-

Table 5: Terms for Red Blood Cell Abnormalities

These conditions can be seen in microscopic examination of blood smears.

Anisocytosis—Variations in size of red blood cells in a specimen.

Basophilic stippling—If the specimen is stained with basic (nonacid, nonalkaline) dye, a blue network appears on the cells. This does not occur if the cells are normal.

Crenated red cells—The cells shrink and the edges appear spiny instead of smooth and rounded.

Cabot rings—A blue ring appears in the cell when a polychromatic stain (such as Wright's stain) is applied.

Howell-Jolly bodies—One or more large, blue granules appear in the cells. These are remnants of nuclei.

Macrocytosis—A type of anisocytosis in which many larger-than-normal red cells are visible.

Microcytosis—Anisocytosis in which many red cells are smaller than normal.

Ovalocytosis—Red cells appear as ovals rather than round discs.

Poikilocytosis—Red cells are varied in shape, instead of all being the same.

Polychromatophilia—The red cells have a blue tinge throughout the cell.

Spherocytosis—The cells are spherical in shape instead of the normal biconcave discs.

vents the conversion of prothrombin into thrombin is added. Measured amounts of calcium and **thromboplastin (THROM boh PLAS tin)**—the substances that convert prothrombin to thrombin—are then added to the specimen. The time required for these substances to clot the specimen is compared to a known standard to determine how well certain coagulation factors are functioning. This test is used when a patient is taking anticoagulant drugs, to monitor the balance of clotting factors and anticlotting factors in the blood.

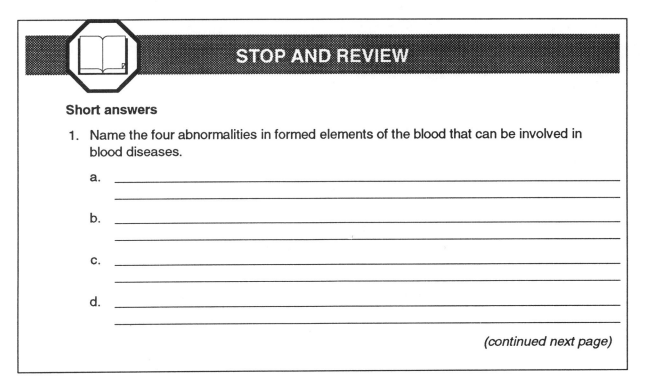

STOP AND REVIEW

Short answers

1. Name the four abnormalities in formed elements of the blood that can be involved in blood diseases.

   a. _____
   _____

   b. _____
   _____

   c. _____
   _____

   d. _____
   _____

(continued next page)

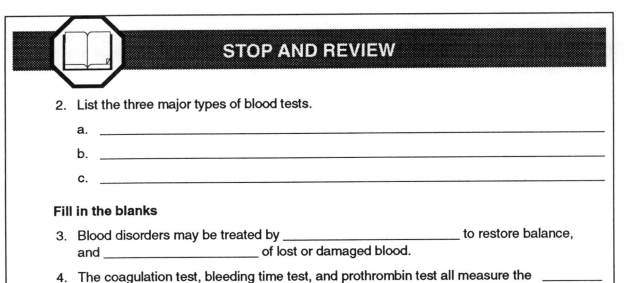

TREATMENT OF BLOOD DISORDERS

Some blood diseases occur as a result of a dietary deficiency, such as inadequate amounts of iron, vitamin B$_{12}$, folic acid, or vitamin K. These diseases are often treated with dietary supplements. In a few cases, the deficiency is due to the patient's inability to digest or absorb a certain nutrient. In such cases, the supplement may have to be given by injection instead of by mouth. Other medications that may be given include anticoagulants or coagulants, antibiotics, steroids, or anticancer (cytotoxic) drugs.

Transfusions may be given in diseases that deplete the supply of formed elements, or when large amounts of blood are lost through injury or major surgery. As we have seen in the section on blood groups in Chapter 1, a transfusion is not merely a matter of replacing lost blood with any available blood. The donor's blood and recipient's blood must be carefully matched. There also are other risks of transfusions besides those of the transfusion reaction. The greatest of these is the risk of contracting an infection such as **hepatitis (HEP ah TYE tis)** or the **acquired immune deficiency syndrome (AIDS)** from the transfused blood. Some infections can be detected in donated blood and thus avoided, but at least one type of hepatitis virus (now known as hepatitis C) cannot be easily detected in donated blood.

The methods and techniques of blood transfusion have become increasingly complex in recent years. It has been discovered that transfusions of whole blood can cause an overload in the patient's circulation, so that currently donated blood is often separated into its components: red cells, platelets, whole plasma, and plasma components such as albumin. Thus, the one specific element needed by the patient can in some cases be provided without the inclusion of unnecessary components. Also, some components are easier to preserve than others. For example, red blood cells can be stored frozen for 1 year or longer.

One other treatment for blood diseases should be mentioned—a surgical treatment, called **splenectomy (splee NECK toh mee)**. In certain forms of anemia, the **spleen**

Fill in the blanks

1. Inadequate amounts of _____, vitamin _____, folic acid, or vitamin _____ in the diet can result in blood diseases.

2. The greatest risks in transfusion are the risks of _____
   and _____ .

3. A surgical treatment for blood diseases is _____, used when the spleen is destroying too many _____ blood cells.

4. Anemia can be defined as _____
   _____ .

becomes overactive in destroying red blood cells; or the number of red cells being destroyed is excessive for some reason. In such cases, removal of the spleen may be necessary. The spleen is not essential to life; this organ can be removed with few adjustment problems for the patient.

BLOOD DISEASES

Iron-Deficiency Anemia

This form of anemia usually is caused by a deficiency of iron in the diet relative to the needs of the body. Some people need to have extra iron in their diets because of extra demands for iron. Examples are pregnant women, and women who regularly have heavy menstrual periods. Some patients who have slow internal bleeding due, for example, to a stomach ulcer, have **iron-deficiency anemia**. Others simply do not take in enough iron for normal needs. In a few cases, iron in the diet is not absorbed by the digestive system.

The symptoms of anemia are paleness, fatigue, weakness, rapid heartbeat or palpitations, and sometimes breathlessness after exertion. The disease is diagnosed by blood tests: measures of hemoglobin and red blood cells, and examination of the red cells for abnormalities such as **microcytosis (MYE kroh sye TOH sis)** or small size, **hypochromia (HYE poh KROH mee ah)** or paleness, **anisocytosis (an IYE soh sye TOH sis)**, and **poikilocytosis (POI kih loh sye TOH sis)**. The amount of iron in the patient's serum may also be measured.

Treatment of iron-deficiency anemia usually consists of taking oral iron supplements until the anemia is resolved. This may require many weeks, depending on the severity of the problem and the dose of iron prescribed. It is usually best to supply the extra iron gradually and allow the body to gradually restore normal levels of red cells and hemoglobin. Sometimes oral iron causes side effects such as abdominal cramps, constipation, or diarrhea. In most cases, reducing the dose relieves these symptoms. It is important to warn patients to keep iron tablets away from children and not to exceed recommended doses. Excess iron can build up to toxic levels in the body and cause severe symptoms or even death.

In a few cases, such as when the problem is caused by malabsorption of iron, the iron can be given by injection. In very severe cases, a transfusion of red blood cells or whole blood may be necessary.

If the problem seems to be caused by an underlying disorder such as internal bleeding or malabsorption, the physician will investigate that disorder and try to resolve it. But treatment for the anemia itself is usually started immediately, regardless of the cause.

Folic Acid-Deficiency Anemia and B₁₂-Deficiency Anemia

These forms of anemia are quite similar to iron-deficiency anemia, except that the missing ingredients are different. **Folic acid-deficiency anemia** is common in pregnancy because the developing fetus requires extra amounts of this nutrient. **Vitamin B₁₂-deficiency anemia** is found most often in alcoholics and others who do not eat a balanced diet. This deficiency may also occur in patients who have had digestive surgery. The symptoms are similar to those of iron-deficiency anemia. However, severe B₁₂ deficiency can also cause neurological symptoms, since this vitamin is important to the function of the nervous system. The patient may have numbness or tingling in the hands and feet and difficulty with walking and balance, and may become confused, depressed, or disoriented. These problems are diagnosed by symptoms, patient history and diet, and blood tests. The treatment is usually supplementation of the missing vitamins by oral or intramuscular methods.

Pernicious Anemia

Pernicious (per NISH us) anemia is a particular form of vitamin B₁₂-deficiency anemia in which the patient receives sufficient vitamin in the diet but cannot absorb it because the stomach lining does not produce intrinsic factor. This substance must be present before the digestive tract can absorb vitamin B₁₂. The symptoms are the same as in other anemias, but oral doses of the vitamin do not affect the condition.

Pernicious anemia cannot be cured. It is treated with injections of the vitamin, which must be given regularly for the patient's lifetime. The body can store vitamin B₁₂, so that once the patient's condition is stabilized by daily injections, a monthly dose can be given. Sometimes the patient or a family member can be taught to give the injections at home.

ANEMIA OF CHRONIC DISEASES

Anemia may occur as a complication of chronic or other serious diseases. Examples are rheumatoid arthritis, hepatitis, tuberculosis, and pneumonia. The symptoms are like those of other anemias: paleness, tiredness, weakness, palpitations. These symptoms sometimes are difficult to distinguish from the symptoms of the underlying disorder. The problem is diagnosed by blood tests. Since the anemia is caused by the original disease, it may not be treatable except by transfusions. Successful treatment of that underlying problem should relieve the anemia as well.

Hemolytic Anemia

Hemolysis (hee MOL ih sis) means destruction of blood cells. In **hemolytic (HEE moh LIT ick) anemia**, red blood cells are destroyed prematurely, and the production of cells in the bone marrow cannot keep up with the rate of cell destruction. In some cases, this is caused by a hereditary abnormality in the blood. One of these inherited abnormalities is **glucose-6-phosphate-dehy-**

drogenase (FOS fayt dee HYE droh jen ays; G6-P-D) deficiency, in which a particular enzyme is missing from the blood. When the patient takes certain drugs or eats certain foods, a reaction occurs and red blood cells are destroyed (hemolyzed) in the blood vessels. Hemolytic anemia can also occur as an autoimmune reaction—the body, for an unkown reason, makes antibodies against its own red blood cells. In other cases, the reason for the hemolysis is not known.

The symptoms of hemolytic anemia are paleness, fatigue, weakness, palpitations, jaundice (yellowing of the skin) and sometimes darker than normal or pink to red urine. It is diagnosed by blood and urine tests. The red cells will probably have an abnormal shape or size, and the hemoglobin level and red cell count will be low. High levels of hemoglobin may be found in the plasma and in the urine. A reticulocyte count may also be useful.

Treatment of the disorder depends on the cause. Any causative drugs will be discontinued, and the physician will advise the patient to avoid foods that cause hemolysis. In some forms of the disease, a splenectomy is recommended to reduce the rate of red cell destruction. This improves the condition but does not cure it. Transfusions may be helpful, but in some cases the donated blood hemolyzes as well, making the situation even worse. In cases where the cause is an autoimmune reaction, steroid drugs may resolve the problem.

Aplastic Anemia

The bone marrow is at the center of the problem of **aplastic (ah PLAS tick) anemia**. The marrow reduces production of all blood cells, thus causing an overall deficit of red cells, granulocytes, and platelets. It can be caused by exposure to toxic chemicals or radioactivity or by a drug prescribed for an unrelated disease, but in many cases the cause in not known.

Aplastic anemia symptoms are those of ordinary anemia plus susceptibility to bacterial infection due to the lack of granulocytes, and symptoms of bleeding disorders. These include a rash consisting of red dots just under the skin, bruising, nosebleeds, bleeding of the gums, and other abnormal bleeding. The problem is diagnosed by blood counts and confirmed by a bone marrow biopsy. The doctor will question the patient about exposure to radiation or chemicals at work, and about drugs the patient is taking. If the problem is caused by one of those, the patient must avoid the exposure or stop taking the drugs. The symptoms are treated with transfusions and antibiotics. In some cases the problem clears up with removal of the cause or with treatment. In other cases the condition worsens. Bone marrow transplants may be helpful in severe cases, if a suitable donor can be found.

There are many other forms of anemia, but those described above are the most common.

Thrombocytopenia

In this disorder, the number of platelets is reduced to one third or more below normal. This can be caused by drug reactions, radiation therapy or chemotherapy prescribed to treat cancer, or an autoimmune reaction with no known cause. It can also be a symptom of leukemia or excessive blood loss.

The symptoms of **thrombocytopenia (THROM boh SYE toh PEE nee ah)** are a rash that looks like small red dots (usually beginning on the legs), nosebleeds, bruising, and sometimes prolonged bleeding from minor cuts. Internal bleeding may also occur. The rash is caused by bleeding from broken

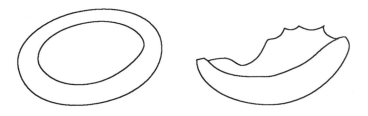

Figure 9: Comparison of normal red blood cell to sickled cell

capillaries under the skin.

The problem is diagnosed by a platelet count, bleeding tests, and sometimes an examination of the bone marrow. Treatment depends on the cause. If drugs are the cause, they will be withdrawn. An autoimmune reaction may be treated with steroid drugs, and may resolve in a few weeks. Splenectomy may be recommended in some cases, as the spleen may become overactive and destroy platelets. In severe cases, platelet transfusions may be necessary.

Sickle Cell Anemia

Sickle cell anemia is an inherited disorder of the red blood cells. It centers around production of an abnormal form of hemoglobin called hemoglobin S. Hemoglobin S differs from normal hemoglobin in that one chemical element is substituted for another in the structure of the molecule. Erythrocytes having this abnormal hemoglobin wear out faster than normal. They also become deformed, taking a sickled shape instead of the normal biconcave disk (see Figure 9). This deformity occurs most often when there is a shortage of oxygen in the body, or in areas of the body that are low in oxygen. The sickled cells are less flexible than normal erythrocytes, and have difficulty passing through small blood vessels. This causes blockages in the capillaries and lack of oxygen in the tis-

sues, which makes the sickling even worse.

Sickle cell anemia is inherited when both parents have the gene for it and both pass it on to the fetus. It is also possible to have only one gene for the disease. This is known as **sickle cell trait**. A person with the trait does not have the disease, but does have the capacity to pass it on to any offspring. This disease is found only in persons of African, Italian, Greek, Arabian, and Indian descent. In the United States, it is most common in the black population; approximately 1 in 1000 black Americans has the disease. The trait is even more common; six of every 1000 black couples could pass the disease to their offspring.

The symptoms of sickle cell anemia are those of ordinary anemia, plus occasional sickle cell crises. In a crisis, large numbers of erythrocytes become sickled due to stress such as an illness or an injury. This causes severe pain in the bones, joints, and abdomen. With each crisis, organs and tissues are damaged by impaired blood flow, and the patient's general health is threatened. Patients also are especially susceptible to infection. These complications can eventually lead to death from a severe infection or organ failure.

The disease is diagnosed by blood tests and family history. An examination of erythrocytes deprived of oxygen will show the characteristic sickled shape. The type of hemoglobin in the cells can then be determined. There is no cure for the disease. Crises are treated with hospitalization and pain-killing drugs. Patients are encouraged to get prompt treatment for even minor injuries and infections to help them avoid crises. Precautions are necessary before any surgery or dental treatment, and situations where there may be a shortage of oxygen, such as high altitude, should be avoided. Anyone who has a family history of the disease should have blood tests done and, if the trait is found, genetic counseling should occur before a family is started.

Thalassemia

Like sickle cell anemia, **thalassemia (THAL ah SEE mee ah)** is inherited and can be carried as a genetic trait without causing symptoms. It also is an abnormality of hemoglobin. In this case, no normal hemoglobin is formed. Instead, small amounts of hemoglobin F, which usually occurs only in newborns, are made as partial compensation. Even those blood cells made with hemoglobin F have a shorter-than-normal lifespan. Some do not leave the bone marrow before they are destroyed. Therefore, the patient with the disease, known as **thalassemia major**, constantly has severe anemia. The symptoms are those of other anemias—paleness, weakness, fatigue, palpitations. These symptoms persist, and restrict activity severely. The patient may also have abnormal bone development if the illness begins in childhood and is not treated promptly.

Thalassemia occurs most often in populations resident near the Mediterranean Sea, in the Middle East, and in the Far East, and their descendants. Like sickle cell anemia, it cannot be cured.

The treatment for thalassemia major is regular blood transfusions. This has a side effect: the build-up of excess iron in the body. A drug is prescribed to eliminate that iron and prevent the toxic effects of build-up. In some cases, removal of the spleen is also helpful. If the disease is severe and transfusions are frequent, the iron may eventually build up to dangerous levels and cause death, even with drug treatment.

Hemophilia

Hemophilia is an inherited clotting disorder. It is inherited almost exclusively by males from female carriers of the trait, because it is a sex-linked characteristic. (See the book on bio-organization in this series for more information about inheritance.)

In hemophilia, the patient has less than the normal supply of a protein called **Factor VIII**, or **antihemophilic (AN tih HEE moh FIL ick) factor**, in the plasma. This protein has an important role in the clotting mechanism, related to the formation of thromboplastin. As a result of this deficiency, minor injuries can cause prolonged and extensive bleeding. Bleeding may also occur in the joints.

The symptoms of hemophilia usually appear first in early childhood. Crawling produces bruises on the baby's knees, and small injuries bleed excessively. The severity of the symptoms varies from patient to patient. In the most severe cases, the joints become stiff from internal bleeding and the limbs swell painfully.

Treatment for hemophilia requires infusions of antihemophilic factor, which can be extracted from pooled donated blood. Hemophiliacs also must limit their activity to try to prevent even the most minor injuries. Special preparation is required before any surgery or dental treatment.

Hereditary Spherocytosis

In this disorder, some of the patient's red blood cells are spherical instead of disk shaped. These abnormal cells are smaller than other red cells, and are uniform in color instead of having a pale center. The condition is inherited.

The spherical erythrocytes are more fragile than normal, and have a lower survival rate than other red cells. The number of these spherical erythrocytes varies considerably among patients, and also with time. In some patients, the disease causes few or no symptoms until a crisis occurs, often precipitated by an infection. The spherocytes are rapidly destroyed, and sudden severe anemia results.

The symptoms of **hereditary spherocytosis (SFEE roh sye TOH sis)** are anemia, jaundice (caused by excess destruction of red cells and resulting in high levels of bilirubin in the blood), and an enlarged spleen. It is diagnosed by examination of the red cells to detect spherocytes, a reticulocyte count (which is higher than normal, especially during crises), and family history.

Treatment may initially involve giving transfusions of red cells, especially in a crisis. The main treatment, however, is splenectomy. For reasons that are not fully understood, removal of the spleen seems to prevent premature hemolysis of the spherocytes.

NEOPLASTIC DISEASES—THE LEUKEMIAS AND MULTIPLE MYELOMA

Leukemia and **multiple myeloma (MYE eh LOH mah)** are cancers of the white blood cells. There are many forms of leukemia. They vary with the type of cell that is affected, and some types are chronic, or long-term, while others are acute, or short-term. Though leukemia is a disease of the white blood cells, other blood cells are affected because abnormal white blood cells disrupt the bone marrow, where other cells are made. Multiple myeloma occurs in the bone marrow, and also has a destructive effect on other blood cells and the bone itself.

Acute Lymphocytic Leukemia

Acute lymphocytic leukemia (LIM foh SIT ick loo KEE mee ah) most often affects children. Some of the lymphocytes become cancerous and multiply excessively. The cause is not known, but the disease is possibly related to exposure to radiation, certain chemicals, certain viruses, and also to heredity. The abnormal cells enter the bloodstream and cause damage to the liver, spleen, bone marrow, and central nervous system. In the bone marrow, they interfere with the manufacture of erythrocytes, platelets, and neutrophils.

The symptoms include anemia that becomes progressively more severe, swollen glands, pain in joints from bleeding, a rash of red dots beneath the skin, an enlarged spleen, susceptibility to infections (especially pneumonia), sores in the mouth and throat, and severe headaches. The disease is diagnosed by bone marrow biopsy and blood tests.

Acute lymphocytic leukemia is often treated in the hospital. The patient is given cytotoxic drugs and steroids to try to eliminate the abnormal blood cells and promote production of normal cells. If the central nervous system is affected, anticancer drugs may be injected into the cerebrospinal fluid. Antibiotics are given intravenously to fight infection, and platelet transfusions may be needed to prevent abnormal bleeding.

Sometimes the child must be kept in isolation to prevent contact with an infected person, since resistance is extremely low during this treatment.

Usually after a few weeks the disease enters **remission (ree MISH un)**. That is, the symptoms disappear and the body resumes normal production of blood cells. This lasts for 5 years or more in about half the cases. In other cases the disease does not respond to treatment, or it returns after a few months or years, and the treatment must be repeated. The more often the disease recurs, the smaller the possibility for complete recovery. Some patients eventually die from the disease.

Acute Myelogenous Leukemia

This form of leukemia mainly affects the granulocytes, in an early stage of development. The earliest forms of granulocytes are called **myeloblasts (MYE eh loh BLASTS)**, and more mature forms are **myelocytes (MYE eh loh syts)**; it is from these forms that the name of the disease is derived. In the bone marrow, immature granulocytes become abnormal. Instead of maturing, they multiply. As their numbers increase, they disrupt production of other blood cells. Abnormal forms of other blood cells may also occur. The abnormal cells then enter the bloodstream and damage organs, including the liver and spleen.

The symptoms are fatigue, infections of the mouth and throat, mouth ulcers, fever, bruising and bleeding, and sometimes the symptoms of anemia. The symptoms usually appear suddenly, and can be fatal shortly thereafter unless the disease is treated. **Acute myelogenous (MYE eh LOJ eh nus) leukemia** is diagnosed by bone marrow biopsy and examination of the blood. The abnormal cells can be seen under a microscope. Once it is diagnosed, the patient is hospitalized for intensive treatment with transfusions, antibiotics, and anticancer drugs. The cancer drugs usually stop most activity in the bone marrow, and about 2 weeks are required for normal levels of normal cells to return to the circulation. During this time the patient is very weak and susceptible to fatal infection. If the treatment is effective, a remission follows. The remission may be lengthy or brief, but this form of leukemia usually returns eventually. It is treated again, and a series of remissions and treatments may follow. The remissions become shorter each time, and the patient eventually dies. About 20 percent of patients live for 5 years or longer after the disease is diagnosed. Bone marrow transplants given during the first remission may prolong the patient's life, and have been responsible for a few cures.

Chronic Lymphocytic Leukemia

This disease usually occurs in adults and develops slowly. It is sometimes several years before the abnormal lymphocytes cause symptoms. The symptoms are swollen glands, enlarged spleen, and sometimes anemia or recurring or persistent infections. Occasionally initial symptoms are more vague: general poor health, loss of appetite, and fever. The disease is diagnosed by examination of the blood to find excessive numbers of lymphocytes, or immature and abnormal lymphocytes. It may be discovered before symptoms are noted, if the patient has a blood test for some other reason.

Treatment of **chronic lymphocytic leukemia** usually is not begun until symptoms begin to appear. An anticancer drug is then prescribed. If it is effective, the symptoms clear and no further treatment is needed until symptoms reappear. Sometimes the usual drug does not work, or stops working after a period of time. Other drugs, usually in combination, are then prescribed and may keep the disease under control for a period of time. In some cases, radiation treatment is also prescribed. Most patients live for 3 to 4 years, and some for up to 15 years, but the disease eventually resists all treatment and results in death.

Chronic Myelogenous (Myeloid) Leukemia

This is a chronic form of myelogenous leukemia. It affects the granulocytic series of cells, causing them to multiply to 20 to 40 times the normal number in the bone marrow. They disrupt production of red blood cells, then enter the bloodstream and cause the spleen and liver to enlarge. The cancerous granulocytes are not as effective against infection as normal cells are, so protection against bacteria is limited.

The symptoms are general poor health, loss of appetite and weight, fever, abnormal sweating at night, enlarged spleen, and symptoms of anemia. Without treatment, the disease usually is fatal within a few months. It is diagnosed by examination of blood and bone marrow. The blood usually contains every stage of immature granulocytes, instead of only mature granulocytes, and a few band cells.

Treatment is with a drug that can be taken on an outpatient basis. Some patients require constant dosing, while others need it only intermittently. However, regular blood tests (every 2 to 4 weeks) are necessary to adjust the dose. Otherwise the number of normal blood cells may fall too low and make the patient weak and susceptible to infection.

Eventually, treatment becomes less effective, and the disease enters a stage that resembles acute leukemia. This is called **acute transformation (TRANS for MAY shun)**. After this occurs, a series of treatments and gradually shorter remissions follow, ending in death.

Multiple Myeloma

Multiple myeloma is cancer of the plasma cells. Plasma cells are derived from B-cells. They produce antibodies to combat viral infections and other foreign material. These cells are made in the bone marrow. When one becomes malignant (cancerous), it multiplies until the excessive number of cells disrupts production of other cells in the marrow. At the same time, plasma cell tumors spread from the marrow, and damage the bone. The remaining normal plasma cells become less effective than usual in producing antibodies, so that the kidneys and the nervous system may be impaired.

The symptoms of multiple myeloma are bone pain (especially the vertebrae), anemia, and susceptibility to infection. Mental confusion and urinary problems may also occur. Destruction of bone can cause high calcium levels in the blood and urine, and kidney damage causes protein to appear in blood and urine. Multiple myeloma is diagnosed by blood and urine tests, examination of the bone marrow, and x-ray studies of the skeleton, to detect the characteristic bone damage.

Treatment includes giving carefully controlled doses of a drug that destroys the malignant cells. The drug may also damage normal cells, so frequent blood tests and protection from infection are necessary. Antibiotics may be prescribed. Radiation treatment may reduce bone pain. Patients are advised to drink extra fluids to improve kidney function. With treatment, the expected survival time for a patient with multiple myeloma is 2 to 3 years, or may be longer. About one third of patients die from a sudden acute phase of the disease, in which treatments suddenly are ineffective.

Polycythemia

Polycythemia (POL ee sye THEE mee ah) is a neoplastic disease, but it is benign rather than malignant. In this disorder the bone marrow overproduces normal erythrocytes, or a combination of erythrocytes, granulocytes, and platelets. **Polycythemia vera (VEE rah)** causes overproduction of all blood cells by the bone marrow. The cause is not known. A condition called secondary polycythemia can occur as an effect of another disorder that limits the oxygen supply, such as a lung or heart disorder. Smoking or living at high altitudes can also cause this form of the disorder. It causes overproduction of red cells only.

The problem is diagnosed by blood counts and other tests to determine which of the diseases is present. Blood volume is estimated and the kidneys are also tested to determine whether the apparent excess of blood cells is being caused by dehydration.

The symptoms of polycythemia vera are headache, dizziness, a feeling of fullness, and flushed skin. The skin may also itch, and the spleen may be enlarged. The excess cells can cause excessive clotting, which may lead to a heart attack (from a clot in the heart), thrombosis, and stroke.

Treatment begins with removal of blood, usually 1 pint at a time, to reduce the number of cells. If necessary, drugs are prescribed also to suppress bone marrow activity. These measures may halt the disease for several years, but treatment may have to be repeated periodically throughout the patient's life, whenever the blood count increases.

Septicemia

Septicemia (SEP tih SEE mee ah) occurs when a bacterial infection, usually but not always caused by **gram-negative bacteria,** enters the bloodstream instead of remaining localized in a specific location or organ. The bacteria in the bloodstream release toxins, or poisons, that can interrupt blood flow and damage tissue and organs. If it is not detected and treated, septicemia can lead to shock and eventually death.

The initial symptoms of septicemia are chills, fever, nausea, vomiting, diarrhea, and prostration. If shock occurs, these symptoms are followed by rapid heartbeat; cold, pale, clammy skin; and cyanosis, a bluish color of the skin. Diagnosis usually is made on the basis of the symptoms in the presence of a known infection. In the elderly or chronically ill patient, however, the symptoms may not be as apparent. An elevated white blood cell count and bacteria in the blood may or may not be present.

Treatment of septicemia with shock requires administration of oxygen; intravenous fluids may be given to increase blood volume; and specific antibiotics are given to treat a specific infection identified by culture. If an organ is abscessed, it may have to be surgically drained and repaired. Other measures such as heart stimulation, opening blood vessels, maintaining urine flow, and eliminating toxins from the blood can be taken through administration of various drugs. These measures are not always successful in reversing septic shock. It is best to detect septicemia early and treat it with appropriate antibiotics before shock occurs.

Matching

1. Mix and match anemia and cause or causes.

    Anemia

    _____ Iron-deficiency   _____ Hemolytic

    _____ Folic-acid deficiency   _____ Aplastic

    _____ B$_{12}$ deficiency   _____ Sickle-cell

    _____ Pernicious

    Cause

    a. Iatrogenic   e. Internal bleeding

    b. Malabsorption   f. Bone marrow inactivity

    c. Pregnancy   g. Hereditary abnormality

    d. Lack of balanced diet   h. Autoimmune reaction

Short answers

2. Thalassemia is like sickle cell anemia because

    a. _____

    b. _____

Fill in the blanks

3. A platelet count is an important tool in diagnosing _____ ,
    a disease in which the number of platelets is greatly reduced.

4. Leukemia affects blood cells other than WBCs because _____.

5. The cause of septicemia is usually a gram-_____ bacterial infection
    that enters the _____ where it releases _____
    that can interrupt blood flow and damage tissues and organs.

(continued next page)

Matching

6. Mix and match neoplastic disease with characteristic.

   Disease

   _____ Acute lymphocytic leukemia

   _____ Acute myelogenous leukemia

   _____ Chronic lymphocytic leukemia

   _____ Chronic myelogenous leukemia

   _____ Multiple myeloma

   _____ Polycythemia

   Characteristic

   a. Benign rather than malignant

   b. Lymphocytes become cancerous

   c. Usually occurs in adults

   d. Affects plasma cells

   e. Immature granulocytes become abnormal

   f. Mature granulocytes multiply to 20–40 times normal amount

   g. Disrupts production of RBCs

   h. Abnormal cells interfere with functions of bone marrow

   i. Tumors develop in bone marrow

   j. Normal forms of erythrocytes, granulocytes, platelets are overproduced

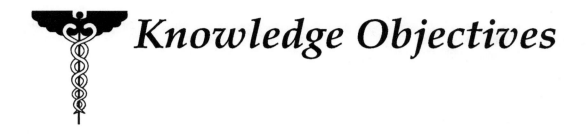

Knowledge Objectives

After completing this chapter, you will be able to:

- describe the structure and function of the lymphatic system
- describe the composition and function of lymph
- describe the composition and function of lymph nodes and lymphatic tissue
- describe the structure and function of the spleen
- describe the structure and function of the thymus
- explain the immune response
- describe the structure and function of the immune system
- explain humoral immunity
- explain cell-mediated immunity
- explain how immunization and vaccination work
- list the five classes of immunoglobulins, and explain their functions

The Anatomy and Physiology of the Lymphatic and Immune Systems

INTRODUCTION

The **lymphatic (lim FAT ick) system**, immune system, and blood intermingle and work together so that sometimes it is hard to tell where one starts and the other stops. It can be argued that the lymphatic system is not a single system but an extension of the cardiovascular system. The blood's leukocytes (white blood cells) provide immunity as they circulate. The immune system defends the body by means of the lymphatic and the cardiovascular systems, which fight foreign invaders. Let us examine the lymphatic system first and go on to the immune system later.

THE LYMPHATIC SYSTEM

Like blood, **lymph (LIMF)** is a fluid that is considered a tissue. It has its own system of vessels that penetrate the intercellular spaces throughout the body and eventually drain into the bloodstream. They run near the vessels of the circulatory system. The lymphatic system has six major functions:

- To drain fluid from the intercellular spaces back into the bloodstream after that fluid has delivered oxygen and nutrients to the cells and picked up waste products;
- To return proteins that have leaked out of the blood vessels to the bloodstream;
- To filter toxins (poisons), debris, and other foreign substances from the fluid before it is returned to the blood;
- To manufacture lymphocytes and monocytes;
- To destroy worn-out or defective red blood cells; and
- To carry fat from the intestines to the blood.

In addition to the network of vessels, the system includes **lymph nodes**; two ducts that collect the filtered lymph and return it to the bloodstream; the spleen; and the thymus.

Lymphatic Vessels

The smallest of the lymph vessels are called **lymph capillaries (KAP ih LAR eez)**, like their counterparts in the circulatory system. They are microscopic, thin-walled tubes that have permeable walls. Through the walls, interstitial fluid moves into the lymphatic system, and, at that point, becomes lymph. Lymph is similar to plasma, except that it contains less protein. Most plasma proteins remain in the blood capillaries, which have less permeable walls than lymph capillaries. Any proteins that do leak out of the blood vessels are picked up by the lymphatic system and returned to the blood. Lymph capillaries are located throughout the body, except in the brain and spinal cord (central nervous system), eyeball and surrounding fat, inside of the ear, cartilage, and epidermis (outermost layer of the skin) (see Figure 10).

The capillaries drain into collecting vessels. These vessels are larger, but still thin walled. They contain valves that prevent lymph from flowing back to the interstitial fluid. Lymph is not pumped through the veins and arteries. Instead, the contraction of smooth muscles along the vessel walls keeps the fluid moving, and the valves keep it from flowing backward between contractions.

The collecting vessels pass through lymph nodes. There the fluid is filtered, and debris, toxins, bacteria, dead cell fragments, and other foreign substances are removed and destroyed. The vessels that enter the nodes are called **afferent (AF er ent) lymphatic vessels**, and those that leave are called **efferent (EF er ent) lymphatic vessels**. The efferent vessels eventually join together to form larger vessels that lead to either the **thoracic (thor RAS ick) duct** or the **right lymphatic duct**.

The thoracic duct (see Figure 10) is the larger of the two ducts, and all the lymph vessels from the left half of the body and the lower part (below the diaphragm) of the right side of the body drain into it. This duct extends from the second lumbar vertebra (between the pelvis and the lowest rib) to the base of the neck, along the spinal column. A widening at the lowest part of the duct is called the **cisterna chyli (sis TER nah KYE lye)**, because it holds **chyle (KYL)**, or lymph permeated with fat.

Chyle comes from the lymph vessels surrounding the intestines. Fats from the digestive system are carried into the bloodstream by the following path: to the lymph capillaries in the intestinal walls, to the collecting vessels, and to the base of the thoracic duct. The duct empties into the junction of the left subclavian vein and the left internal jugular vein, in the base of the neck.

The right lymphatic duct (see Figure 10) is the smaller of the two lymph ducts. It is located between the base of the neck and the first rib, opposite the apex (top) of the thoracic duct. It empties into the right **brachycephalic (BRACK ee oh seh FAL ick) vein**. Many people do not have this duct. If it is not present, collecting vessels from the upper right section of the body drain directly into the right brachycephalic vein.

Lymph Nodes and Lymphatic Tissue

Lymphatic tissue is a mesh of fibrous tissue that contains hematopoietic stem cells, the cells from which blood cells are made. This tissue is found at strategic locations around the body, in the form of either **nodules** or

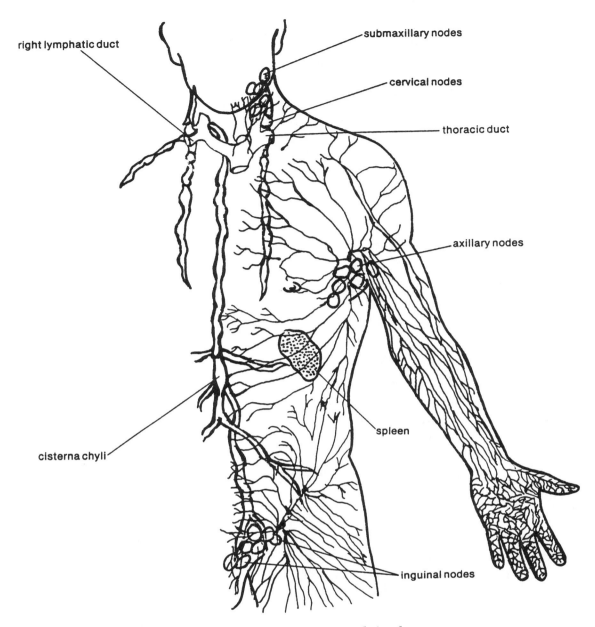

right lymphatic duct

submaxillary nodes

cervical nodes

thoracic duct

axillary nodes

spleen

cisterna chyli

inguinal nodes

Figure 10: The lymphatic system, including lymph nodes, speen, and circulatory systems

nodes. Nodules are smaller than nodes. They are found in areas of the body that are regularly exposed to contamination from outside, such as the inner lining of the digestive system, the respiratory system, and the urinary tract.

Lymph nodes are found in clusters along the lymphatic vessels. They are oval structures of varying sizes (up to the size of an almond), made of lymphatic tissue and divided into compartments called germinal centers (Figure 11). In these compartments, hematopoietic cells make lymphocytes. The lymphocytes are released into a network of **sinuses**, or channels, that surround the compartments. In these sinuses, fibers form nets

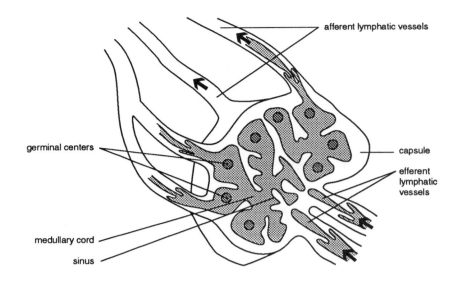

Figure 11: Structure of a lymph node

to which cling reticuloendothelial cells. As lymph passes though the sinuses, these nets filter the fluid and remove foreign particles. Sometimes, when an infection is present, bacteria or viruses accumulate in large numbers in the lymph nodes, causing them to become inflamed. This is called **swollen glands.** The medical terms for it are **lymphadenitis (lim FAD eh NYE tis)** and **lymphadenopathy (lim FAD eh NOP ah thee).**

The four major clusters of lymph nodes called regional lymph nodes are:

- **Cervical (SER vih kal) nodes,** which are located in the neck;
- **Submaxillary (sub MACK sih LER ee) nodes,** located in the floor of the mouth;

- **Axillary (ACK sih LAR ee) nodes,** located in the armpits (axillae); and
- **Inguinal (ING gwih nal) nodes,** located in the groin.

THE SPREAD OF CANCER THROUGH THE LYMPHATICS

The lymphatic system provides an effective system for drainage, recycling, and filtering of body fluids. The lymph nodes play an immunological role in controlling cancer, and also act as filters, delaying and interfering with the spread of cancer cells. However, when the filter in the lymph node is overwhelmed with cancer cells, the cancer will spread from one site to another via the lymphatic system. During cancer surgery, these malignant lymph nodes are removed and their vessels are cut off and tied to prevent the further spread of malignant cells. Cancer that migrates from a primary site to another site (often through the lymphatic system) is known as metastatic (MET ah STAT ick) cancer.

Another well-known cluster of lymphatic tissue (actually neither nodules nor nodes) is the **tonsils**. There are three sets of tonsils, the **pharyngeal (fah RIN jee al), lingual (LIN gwal)**, and **palatine (PAL ah tyn)**. In childhood, these form a protective ring around the apex (top) of the pharynx, or throat, to prevent severe infection from penetrating the lungs. The tonsils themselves often become infected in childhood. In most adults they gradually shrink.

The Spleen

The spleen is located beside the stomach, just below the diaphragm (see Figure 10). It is made up of lymphatic tissue, with a covering and framework of connective tissue and smooth muscle fibers. The framework supports two types of material called **splenic (SPLEN ick) pulp**—red splenic pulp and white splenic pulp. The bulk of the spleen is made of red pulp. The white pulp is found in nodules throughout the organ. The white pulp is the site of lymphocyte production in the spleen.

In the red pulp, blood leaves the blood vessels and flows through a network of fibers similar to that found in the sinuses of the lymph nodes. This network contains red blood cells, lymphocytes, and reticuloendothelial cells. Here, defective red blood cells and foreign particles are filtered out and destroyed. The blood returns to the portal vein after this process is completed, and is conveyed to the liver. The spleen extracts iron and **bilirubin (BIL iye ROO bin)** from the red blood cells, and these substances go on to the liver in the blood. In the liver, iron is stored and sent to the bone marrow as needed to make new red blood cells. Bilirubin is eliminated in the **bile**.

During heavy loss of blood, the spleen can add up to 1 pint of blood by emptying its blood into the circulatory system. In a fetus the spleen is the major source of red blood cells. After birth, that function is taken over by the bone marrow.

The Thymus

The thymus is made up of lymphatic tissue located in the lower part of the neck and the upper thorax (chest). It has two pyramidal lobes divided into many smaller sections called lobules. These each have two sections: a medulla, or core, surrounded by a cortex, or outer cover. Each cortex contains many small lymphocytes, and each medulla contains thymic corpuscles, or cell nests.

The thymus enlarges until the child reaches puberty and after puberty it gradually shrinks. Its function is to prepare, or program, lymphocytes to become T-cells, which provide a form of body defense. This process is stimulated by a hormone, thymosin, which is made by the thymus.

At birth, an infant has only limited immunity to disease which is supplied by antibodies from the mother's bloodstream. In the thymus, some of the T-cells develop to regulate production of antibodies that combat diseases as the child becomes exposed to them.

Within a few years, the child has encountered most of the usual infections within the environment, and has manufactured antibodies to combat them. By puberty, the few new agents of infection a person will encounter can be combatted by the accumulated antibodies or by antibodies developed within in the immune system. At this point, the thymus begins to atrophy or become smaller.

STOP AND REVIEW

Short answers

1. Name the six functions of the lymphatic system.

   a. _____

   b. _____

   c. _____

   d. _____

   e. _____

   f. _____

2. The parts of the lymphatic system.

   a. _____

   b. _____

   c. _____

   d. _____

   e. _____

3. Identify the four clusters of lymph nodes.

   a. _____

   b. _____

   c. _____

   d. _____

Fill in the blanks

4. Cells in the lymphatic system that supplement the work of the WBCs are called _____ cells.

5. Lymph capillaries are like blood capillaries because they too have _____.

6. Of the four clusters of lymph nodes, _____ (how many) are located above the waist.

7. A cluster of lymphatic tissue that is neither nodules nor nodes is the _____.

8. The spleen is composed of _____ tissue, covered and with a frame-work of_____ tissue and _____ fibers.

9. The bulk of the spleen is composed of _____; _____ is found in the nodules throughout the organ.

10. Lymphocytes are produced in the _____ of the spleen.

11. Defective red blood cells and foreign particles are filtered out of the blood in the _____ of the spleen.

12. The function of the thymus before puberty is to _____.

THE IMMUNE SYSTEM

Introduction

The body can defend itself against many foreign invader substances called antigens. It recognizes and eliminates alien cells that enter it, whether they are actually harmful or not. This capability is called the **immune response**. The immune response can be **nonspecific** (generalized reactions against all types of foreign materials) or **specific** (protective reactions against specific antigens). Immune responses can also be innate or acquired. Examples of innate immunity include nonspecific responses such as the skin, acid enzymes in the stomach, and phagocytosis. Acquired responses are more specific in which substances called antibodies and **activated lymphocytes** are produced to fight specific antigens.

Antigens

An antigen can be any cell that excites the immune system to cause a response. A virus, a toxin, a particular foreign protein such as the protein on red blood cells, or a normally harmless particle such a grain of pollen or a flake of animal dander can act as an antigen. Proteins are the strongest antigens. Since proteins are the building blocks of the body, the body must "recognize" its own protein as native and not foreign. The body does, however, recognize another body's protein as an antigen. This response explains why bodies reject transplants from other bodies unless precautions have been taken to limit or deactivate the immune response.

Nonspecific Immune Response

Nonspecific immunity includes a wide range of reactions of several body systems against all types of foreign materials. The function of nonspecific immunity is to limit the entry of antigens, prevent the spread of the antigens, and strengthen the body's immune system. Nonspecific immunity includes responses from the mucous membranes lining various structures, phagocytes and natural killer cells, the inflammatory response, and the secretion of antimicrobrial substances such as complement and **interferon (IN ter FEER on)**, which defend the body against nonspecific invasion.

Secretions of the Mucous Membranes and Other Glands. The skin itself acts as the first defense against outside invaders, with its acidic pH and secretion of sebum, an oily substance toxic to harmful bacteria. (These functions are discussed in the book on dermatology in this series.) The mucous membranes, the sudoriferous (sweat) glands, the sebaceous glands, the lacrimal glands (tear glands) all secrete substances that are potentially harmful to infectious agents. The flow of these fluids cleans skin surfaces and the linings of the respiratory and digestive tracts (see Figure 12), moving potentially harmful substances and irritants through the body and eliminating them. Also, stomach acid kills many potentially harmful bacteria. These mechanisms involve immune system cells and mechanical means to provide a first line of defense at the body's portals—its openings—where it is susceptible to invasion from outside.

Phagocytes and Natural Killer Cells.
Phagocytes and natural killer cells were described in the discussions of white blood cells and the lymphatic system. These include the reticuloendothelial (RE) cells and granulocytes, which phagocytose foreign material and dead cells. Granulocytes move through the body and RE cells remain stationary. Natural killer cells can defend

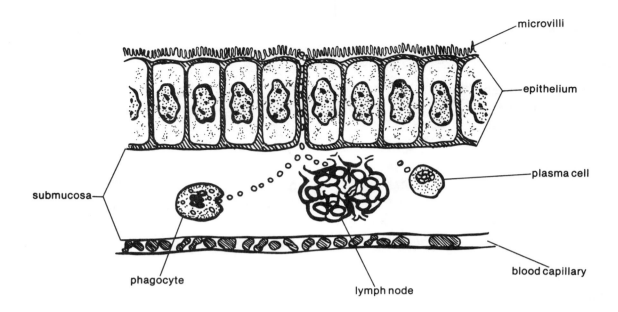

Figure 12: This diagram shows some protective mechanisms to be found in the intestine.

against any antigen, unlike lymphocytes of the immune system, which react to very specific cells.

Inflammatory Response. The inflammatory response has been discussed in the book on bio-organization in this series and earlier in this chapter in the section on blood functions. The increased blood flow and vascular permeability, which develop during the inflammatory response, produce the symptoms of redness, heat, and swelling at the site of infection. The injury is recognized by the body as a form of stress, and nonspecific internal defense systems go into action immediately.

Chemical substances, mostly enzymes and hormones, are released in response to tissue damage. These substances (1) cause blood vessels to dilate, increasing the blood flow; (2) bring phagocytes and leukocytes to the involved area; and (3) start the pain response. Histamine increases vascular permeability, allowing fluids such as plasma, white blood cells, fibrin, and complement to enter the tissues and to cause swelling. Complement in the tissue accelerates the inflammatory process.

The process of increasing the numbers of chemical substances and attracting phagocytes continues until the bacteria are destroyed. Once the causative bacteria have been destroyed, the white blood cells clear the site of infection.

Antimicrobial Substances, Complement and Interferon. In addition to antimicrobrial substances that are secreted during the inflammatory response, histamine, complement, and interferon play the most important roles. There are 11 components of complement proteins in the blood. Complements attach to antigens and can create "holes" in the antigen's surface, causing the cell to lyse, or burst. Complement also speeds up the inflammatory response.

Interferon is a protein produced by most virus-infected cells which interferes with the ability of the virus to reproduce in surrounding cells. Interferon viral resistance acts against many varieties of viruses. Because some cancers are caused by viruses, interferon has been effective in treating them.

Specific Immune Response

The specific immune response protects against specific diseases by destroying or deactivating invading antigens with its antibodies. It is more specialized than the nonspecific immune response. The immune system forms the center of the body's specific immune response.

THE IMMUNE SYSTEM PHYSIOLOGY

The immune system is a functional body system that identifies antigens and deactivates and eliminates them. The body produces substances called antibodies and activated lymphocytes to fight the antigen. Two types of acquired immunity are at work in the immune system: **humoral (HYOO mor al) immunity** and **cell-mediated (SEL MEE dee AY ted) immunity**. Humoral immunity refers to antibodies functioning in the "humors" or fluids of the body. Cell-mediated immunity refers to immunity that is provided when lymphocytes activate to fight antigens. Before discussing humoral immunity and cell-mediated immunity, let us discuss some of the cells that start the immune responses and destroy specific invading cells—lymphocytes and macrophages.

Lymphocytes

Two types of lymphocytes supply immunity when activated: the T- and B-lymphocytes. Both are produced in the red blood marrow. After becoming immunosensitized during fetal development, both types migrate to the lymph nodes and the spleen and other loose connective tissues where their defense against antigens begins.

B-lymphocytes (B-cells) produce antibodies and control humoral immunity. T-lymphocytes (T-cells) do not produce antibodies, but upon being activated by an antigen, they reproduce sensitized T-cells that enter the bloodstream through the lymphatic system. T-cells direct cell-mediated immunity. The antibodies produced by B-cells and th-sensitized T-cells are specifically targeted toward the particular type of antigen for which they were produced.

B-Cells. B-cells were first found in lymph tissue in a digestive organ of birds called the bursa of Fabricius. That is why they are called B-cells. It is believed that the equivalent of the bursa in the human body is the bone marrow. When B-cells are activated by antigens, they begin to produce antibodies, their main function in the immune system.

Some B-cells are transformed into plasma cells, which divide rapidly to produce large numbers of antibodies that are secreted into the lymph and circulated through the bloodstream. Other activated B-cells, called **memory cells**, do not become plasma cells but remain dormant until confronted with the same antigen again. When a memory cell is reactivated by its antigen, the response is quite rapid and produces more antibodies lasting for a longer time than the first exposure to the antigen.

T-Cells. They are called T-cells because during their development they move to the thymus where they are processed for immunization sensitivity. There are several T-cells with different functions: **killer T-cells, helper T-cells, memory T-cells and suppressor T-cells.**

Killer T-cells are activated T-cells capable of killing foreign invaders. Helper T-cells

Table 6: Five Immunoglobulins, Location, and Function

	Where Found	Function
IgG	Plasma; most abundant Ig	Provide passive immunity to newborn by crossing placenta; main antibody for all immune responses.
IgM	Plasma; attached to B-cell	React to foreign red blood cells and foreign tissue; first Ig released by plasma.
IgA	Mucus and excretions in respiratory, and digestive tracts, tears, saliva	Assist in nonspecific immunity against antigens in mucous membranes; prevent microorganisms from attaching to epithelial cells.
IgD	Attached to B-cell	Probably a surface receptor of B-cell, which helps it activate.
IgE	Secreted by plasma cells of skin and mucous membranes	Helps cause the allergic response by binding with the allergen and releasing histamines.

stimulate plasma cells from B-cells to produce larger numbers of antibodies. Suppressor T-cells suppress antibody production by plasma cells and counteract the effect of helper T-cells, normally when a disease has been defeated and it is time for the "troops to go home." Memory T-cells can be any type of T-cell that remains to provide immunologic memory for each antigen.

Antibodies, or Immunoglobulins

Antibodies, or **immunoglobulins (IM yoo noh GLOB yoo linz)** or Ig, are blood plasma proteins that are secreted by activated B-cells, more specifically, plasma cells. Antibodies can bind specifically with the offending antigen. There are five types of Ig, each denoted by Ig followed by a capital letter: **IgG, IgA, IgM, IgD,** and **IgE.** Table 6 describes each of these and its function.

Macrophages

The word macrophage means "big eater." Like B-cells and T-cells, macrophages are formed in bone marrow and are scattered throughout lymph nodes and connective tissues throughout the body. Macrophages swallow and digest antigens and then dis-

play parts of them on their cell surface, to be recognized by T-cells.

Now that we have discussed the cells of the immune system army, we can discuss the two types of acquired immunity—humoral immunity and cell-mediated immunity.

Humoral or Antibody-Mediated Immunity

Humoral or antibody-mediated immunity is immunity provided by antibodies within the body fluids. Humoral immunity can be both **active** and **passive immunity.**

Active immunity can be acquired by receipt of a **vaccine (VACK seen)** or naturally acquired through contact with bacteria or a virus during infections. The immune response is the same either way. However, once the immunity is acquired, the secondary response against the same antigen is much more powerful, due to memory cells.

Most **vaccinations (VACK sih NAY shunz)** include dead or very weakened antigens for a particular disease. Vaccines help us because we do not develop most of the symptoms of the disease from a vaccination and because the weakened antigens stimulate antibody production and promote memory cell production. There may be a mild

Table 7: Immunization Recommendations for Children.

Age	Vaccine
2 months	DPT vaccine (diphtheria toxoid, pertussis (whooping cough) vaccine, and tetanus toxoid), OPV (oral poliomyelitis vaccine)
4 months	DPT vaccine; OPV
6 months	DPT vaccine; (OPV optional for areas with high risk of polio exposure)
15 months	DPT vaccine; OPV; MMR vaccine (combined mumps vaccine, measles vaccine, and rubella virus vaccine) or individual mumps, measles, and rubella virus vaccines. Complete primary series of DPT and OPV
4 to 6 years	DPT vaccine; OPV (preferably at or before school entry)
14 to 16 years	Td vaccine (tetanus and diphtheria toxoid); repeat every 10 years throughout life

reaction such as slight fever or a skin reaction at the site where the vaccine was introduced. In rare cases, the person becomes seriously ill.

"Booster" shots may be given to strengthen the immune response after the first vaccination. Vaccines against pneumonia, smallpox, poliomyelitus (polio), rabies, and diphtheria are available. Parents are advised to have their children immunized against the potentially serious childhood diseases (see Table 7). A vaccinated person has active immunity which has been acquired artificially.

Passive immunity, which is temporary (see Figure 13), occurs when antibodies are acquired from the serum of an immune animal or human. Memory cells do not form, so the temporary protection ends when the antibodies disintegrate in the body. Infants who have received antibodies naturally from their mothers have passive immunity until their own immune system matures sufficiently. Mother's milk also gives the newborn passive immunity.

Cell-Mediated Immunity

Cell-mediated immunity invokes the T-cells to fight targeted foreign invaders. Unlike B-cells, the T-cells do not bind with antigens. T-cells destroy the antigen after the antigen has been digested and excreted by macrophages. Without the macrophage, the T-cell would

ARTIFICIALLY ACQUIRED IMMUNITY

Edward Jenner, an English physician, is credited with the development of vaccination as a preventive against smallpox. Jenner observed that dairy maids who had contracted cowpox were immune to smallpox. In 1796 he encountered a dairy maid who had fresh cowpox lesions on her fingers. Using the matter he scraped from these lesions, he inoculated a small boy with cowpox. The boy developed a slight fever and a low-grade lesion. (Cowpox is an infectious disease caused by a virus closely related to the smallpox virus. In humans, cowpox is not highly severe.) At a later time, Jenner inoculated the boy again, this time with the smallpox virus. The boy did not become ill. Jenner published a paper describing his observations, and a year later vaccinations were introduced into a prominent English hospital. Some time after this, vaccinations were utilized by the English army, navy, and finally the country as a whole.

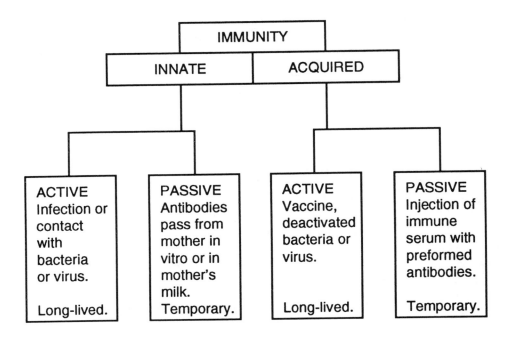

Figure 13: Types of immunity

not recognize the antigen. Once they attach themselves to the digested antigen product, the T-cells release four substances: **cytotoxic (SYE toh TOCK sick) substances** that destroy the antigen product directly; **transfer factor,** which causes nonsensitized lymphocytes at the invasion site to act like sensitized T-cells; **macrophage chemotactic (KEE moh TACK tick) factor,** which attacts additional macrophages to the site; and **macrophage activating factor (MAF),** which increases the phagocytic activity of macrophages.

To aid in their fight against antigens, both macrophages and T-cells produce substances to enhance their performance. **Lymphokines (LIM foh kynz)** are produced by helper T-cells. These substances have vari-

ous functions, one of which is to attract macrophages and convert them to **killer macrophages,** which destroy all surrounding cells whether foreign or not in an attempt to eliminate the antigen. Macrophages secrete proteins called **monokines (MON oh kynz),** which stimulate T-cells to reproduce and cause fever.

Cell-mediated immunity has a regulatory function within the immune system. It stimulates and suppresses activities of the other components of the system. It works more slowly than the humoral system, and normally in a close partnership with that system. As you have seen by the description of several types of T-cells, their action is deadly to the specific antigen they attach.

Fill in the blanks

1. The capability of one body system to recognize and eliminate or destroy foreign substances that enter the body is called the _____; the system that has this capability is the _____ .

2. The two major divisions of the immune system are the _____ , which deals with all types of foreign material, and the _____ component, which responds only to particular antigens.

3. The specific immune response protects the body against specific disease by

    _____ .

4. The immune system produces _____ and _____ to fight against foreign invaders.

5. The type of immunity in which antibodies work in the body fluids is called _____ .

True or False

6. Immune responses can be innate or acquired. T/F

7. Acquired immune responses are present at birth. T/F

8. Passive immune response may be present at birth. T/F

9. Proteins are the strongest antigens. T/F

10. Nonspecific immunity targets specific antigens. T/ F

11. Passive immunity is temporary. T/ F

Matching

12. Write T or B beside each characteristic to indicate whether it is found in T-cells or B-cells.

    ____Produce antibodies

    ____Do not produce antibodies

    ____Direct cell-mediated immunity

    ____Are transformed into plasma cells

    ____Control humoral immunity

    ____Secrete lymph

    ____Are processed in the thymus

    ____Need macrophages to recognize specific antigens

(continued next page)

STOP AND REVIEW

Short answers

13. What type of cell engulfs and digests antigens and then presents them on its outer membrane to the T-cell for destruction? The word means "big eater."

14. List two benefits of being vaccinated with weakened antigens.

    a. _____

    b. _____

Circle the correct answer

15. The response of a memory cell is weaker/stronger the second time it confronts a specific antigen.

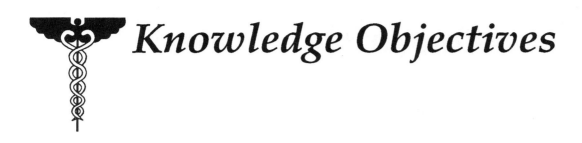
Knowledge Objectives

After completing this chapter, you should be able to:

- list the laboratory tests used in the diagnosis of diseases of the immune system
- describe the causes and treatment of some diseases of the immune system
- describe the causes and treatment of some immunodeficiencies
- describe the causes and treatment of some neoplastic diseases of the lymphatic system
- describe the cause and prevention of AIDS
- describe the cause and treatment of some autoimmune disorders

Diseases of the Lymphatic and Immune Systems

INTRODUCTION

Since the body depends on the lymphatic and immune systems for protection against disease, diseases of these systems can affect the entire body. Often disorders in the lymphatic and immune systems are interdependent and a disease in one affects the other.

Some diseases described here may be symptoms of other diseases rather than diseases in themselves. Examples are **immunodeficiencies (IM yoo noh deh FISH en seez)**, lymphadenopathy, and **leukopenia (LOO koh PEE nee ah)**. They are described here partly to show the interrelationships between these systems and the body as a whole.

DISEASES OF THE LYMPHATIC SYSTEM

Diagnosis and Treatment

Enlargement of the nodes close to the skin can be seen or felt, but enlargement of those inside the body cannot be detected except by x-rays, ultrasound scans, magnetic resonance imaging (MRI), or computed tomography (CT) scans. Enlargement may be suspected based on the results of blood tests,

cultures, biopsies, and other studies.

Cancers of the lymphatic system are diagnosed by biopsy, a laboratory examination of tissue removed from the involved site. Lymph nodes or bone marrow may be biopsied. Treatment for such cancers is with radiation, anticancer drugs, surgery, or a combination of them, and is becoming increasingly successful. It often does have a side effect, however—immune system suppression. The patient must avoid infection while immunity is diminished temporarily, for the anticancer treatment to be effective.

Lymphadenopathy (Swollen Lymph Nodes)

Lymph nodes become swollen, or enlarged, for a number of reasons. In children, swollen glands often occur in mild infections. In adults, this is less common. The nodes swell when infection or inflammation causes them to produce extra lymphocytes, or when they are invaded by abnormal cells either from within or from another source. Lymphadenopathy is a possible symptom of the following disorders: bacterial infections, including staphylococcal, streptococcal, tuberculosis, syphilis, and others; viral infections, including mononucleosis and hepatitis; rheumatoid arthritis and other inflammatory diseases of connective tissue; leukemia; other cancers such as cancer of the breast, lung, head and neck, or kidney; lymphomas; hyperthyroidism; Addison's disease (disorder caused by adrenal gland dysfunction); and diseases of the lymph nodes themselves.

The nodes may be painless, tender, or quite painful. The problem may be accompanied by various symptoms including fever, chills, anemia, coughing, abdominal pain, and others.

Hodgkin's Disease

Hodgkin's (HOJ kinz) disease is a particular form of **lymphoma (lim FOH mah),** or malignant lymphatic tumor. It is distinguished from other lymphomas by a characteristic cell, called a **Reed-Sternberg cell,** which is found in the affected tissue. The disease spreads, either quickly or slowly, first to adjacent lymph nodes, then to more distant nodes, and finally to other organs. The severity of the disease is estimated by its extent and by whether or not the patient has systemic symptoms such as weight loss, fevers, and night sweating. Those with systemic symptoms have less possibility of cure.

Most patients come to the doctor because they have noticed swollen lymph nodes. The nodes are not tender, but they may displace structures around them and cause pain. In later stages, the systemic symptoms mentioned, as well as enlarged liver and spleen,

INFECTED NODULES

When the lymphocytes in the lymph nodes cannot conquer an infection the nodules may become infected. Two common forms of infected nodules are tonsillitis (TON sih LYE tis) and appendicitis (ah PEN dih SYE tis). The tonsils are the first line of defense against any bacterial infection of the pharyngeal walls. Once they are removed, the bacteria may not be detected until the person develops a severe infection. Tonsillitis is a recurring bacterial infection of the pharyngeal tonsils. The person develops a high fever and has an elevated white blood cell count. The tonsils may become inflamed and swollen. With further swelling, swallowing and even breathing may become difficult. As the infection develops, abscesses within the tissue may occur, and the bacteria may enter the bloodstream.

In the early stages of infection, antibiotics may be sufficient treatment. However, once the tonsils have developed abscesses, these must be surgically drained. Recurrent tonsillitis is treated surgically by removing the tonsils, a procedure called tonsillectomy (TON sih LECK toh mee). At one time, tonsillectomies were done routinely in tonsillitis, but this no longer is the case.

The appendix, a blind pouch that originates at the junction of the large and small intestines, also contains a mass of lymphatic tissue. Appendicitis results from the wearing away of the lining of the appendix. This may be due to viral pathogens. Once the appendix becomes infected, it swells and increases its mucus production. Eventually this may cause a rupture, releasing bacteria into the abdominal cavity. Appendicitis is treated by surgically removing the organ, a procedure known as appendectomy (AP en DECK toh mee).

may occur. Diagnosis is made by biopsy of affected tissue.

Treatment depends on the stage the disease has reached at diagnosis. Before the disease has spread, radiation therapy often cures it completely. When the disease is more advanced, a combination of anticancer drugs may produce a remission that may last for up to 15 years.

A few patients who do not respond to initial treatment or who are in the most advanced stages may benefit from a combination of radiation and chemotherapy. After initial successful treatment, patients are monitored for signs of relapse. After a remission, treatment is with drugs rather than radiation. With treatment, about 70 percent of patients recover completely.

Lymphomas (Non-Hodgkin's Lymphomas)

A lymphoma is a malignant tumor of the lymph nodes or lymph tissue. There are many varied lymphomas, differentiated by the type of lymphatic cell that is affected and the appearance of the malignant cells. These tumors can arise anywhere in the body, since lymphatic tissue occurs throughout the body. The disease may spread from the original site to other lymph nodes and other tissues and organs.

The first symptom is usually swollen but painless lymph nodes. Some patients have fever, weight loss for no apparent reason, and symptoms related to growths in other organs. The disease is diagnosed by a biopsy of affected lymph tissue. A number of tests are done once the problem is diagnosed, to determine whether or not the cancer has spread, and its extent. A complete physical examination, additional biopsies, and one or more CT scans may be needed to detect other tumors. The stage of the disease often determines the treatment that the physician will recommend. Radiation treatment and chemotherapy with anticancer drugs, either in combination or alone, are prescribed. Some patients do not require treatment of any sort at first.

Lymphomas are frequently cured. Even if they are not, but if treatment is started early, patients may live for 5 or even 10 years after the diagnosis is made. Eventually, however, treatment loses its effectiveness, and the patient dies. Some patients die of unrelated causes, especially those who are older in the early stage of disease.

Hypersplenism

Either for no known reason or because of another disease process, the spleen sometimes become hyperactive. It may enlarge, and it destroys excessive amounts of blood cells of all types. The signs of the disorder are a spleen that is frequently sufficiently enlarged that a physician (or other trained person) can feel it, and some degree of anemia, abnormal bleeding, and/or immune deficiency from the depletion of blood cells.

To diagnose **hypersplenism (HYE per SPLEEN izm)**, tests measure the rate at which red cells or platelets are being destroyed, and determine where they are being destroyed (whether in the spleen or the liver). If the physician diagnoses hypersplenism, the spleen is sometimes removed. Any underlying cause is treated, which may alleviate the condition.

Ruptured Spleen

Occasionally the spleen will rupture due to an accident or, in rare cases, as the result of a severe infection that causes the spleen to enlarge beyond its capacity to stretch. The rupture causes severe pain in the left upper quadrant of the abdomen, followed by anemia and shock due to internal hemorrhage. When this occurs, the spleen must be removed surgically at once.

IMMUNE SYSTEM DISORDERS AND DISEASES

Diagnosis and Treatment

Sophisticated laboratory tests are necessary to analyze the health of a patient's immune system and defenses against infection. Most related problems can be diagnosed through a combination of the following tests:

- Blood cell count;
- Differential white blood cell count;
- Measures of immunoglobulin levels;
- Tests of T-cell function, for common antibodies and toxins;
- Response to immunization;
- Tests of T-cell function, including skin tests, for reaction, and a chest x-ray film to evaluate the thymus;
- Complement tests, including complement fixation tests and other serological tests; and
- Tests of phagocytic activity.

Treatment usually requires isolation or at least protection of the patient against infection. Sometimes gamma globulin, which contains antibodies extracted from human blood, can be injected to temporarily strengthen the patient's immune system. Some immunity disorders, however, cannot be cured or treated with any notable success.

Immunodeficiencies

Deficiencies of factors in the immune system range from mild and treatable to severe and fatal. Some of these deficiencies are inherited, some are caused by other disease, and some have no known cause. The major sign of such disorders is susceptibility to certain types of infections, which correspond to the immune factor that is depressed or absent.

Immunodeficiency problems are diagnosed by a history of infection and by blood tests that evaluate the presence of immunoglobulins and other immune factors such as T-cells and B-cells. Some deficiencies can be treated by replacing the missing factors. For example, gamma globulin can be extracted from human blood and injected into the patient periodically. In some cases, a child with a deficiency will begin to produce the missing factor at a later time. Specific bacterial infections can be treated with anti-

biotics. When multiple immune factors are missing, however, the patient eventually develops an untreatable infection, and dies. The life span will depend on the number of missing factors and exposure to disease.

Immune deficiency may be an **iatrogenic (eye AT tro JEN ick) disease;** that is, caused by medical treatment. This is expected and guarded against in some cases, as in treatment for leukemia or after an organ transplantation when the immune system is deliberately depressed to prevent rejection of the new organ. Occasionally it occurs as an unexpected side effect of a drug.

Whatever the cause, treatment is aimed at protecting the patient from infection, sometimes by putting him or her in isolation in a hospital, in as sterile an environment as possible. The deficiency is then corrected as soon as conditions allow, usually by discontinuing causative treatments. In some cases, however, the treatment must be continued for some time even when the patient's susceptibility to infection remains extreme, because of the risks involved in discontinuing that treatment.

Allergies

In allergies, the antigen is known as an **allergen (AL er jen).** It is harmless to some individuals, but causes a reaction in others. In allergic reactions, usually there is a mild reaction with the first exposure to the allergen, then more violent reactions thereafter. In sensitive people (those with allergies), exposure to a usually harmless substance such as pollen, dander, feathers, or the oil on certain plant leaves, causes a reaction such as inflammation of the respiratory system or a skin rash. Allergies such as hay fever and other forms of allergic rhinitis and sensitivity to poison ivy are not dangerous, but merely irritating. Other allergies, such as severe reactions to drugs or bee stings, can

BLOOD TRANSFUSION REACTIONS

Blood transfusion reactions are all treated initially the same way: by stopping the transfusion. They can be classified as immunological or nonimmunological. The immunological responses include hemolytic, allergic, and febrile responses. Hemolytic responses occur most often in ABO-incompatible blood. When this happens, the antibodies in the patient's serum react with the donor's RBC antigens. This produces agglutination of the cells which obstructs capillaries and blood flow. Hemolysis of the RBCs releases their hemoglobin into the plasma, which is filtered by the kidneys and found in the urine. Hemoglobin in the renal tubules can lead to acute renal failure.

Hemolytic reactions are usually apparent within the first 15 minutes of beginning the transfusion. They can also be delayed however, appearing 2 to 14 days after the transfusion.

Allergic reactions occur because the recipient is sensitive to a component of the donor's blood. This is seen most often in patients with a history of allergies. The symptoms of allergic reaction include uticaria (hives), itching, edema, or more rarely, swelling of the throat, pulmonary edema, or anaphylaxis (AN ah fih LACK sis). Antihistamines are given immediately. Patients with a history of allergies have fewer problems with washed or leukocyte-depleted RBCs.

Leukocyte and thrombocyte incompatibility is the most common cause of febrile reactions. It is usually brought about by previous transfusions; the recipient's antibodies react with the donor's platelets. Patients usually complains of fever and chills about 1 hour after the transfusion has started. They may complain of headache, flushing, rapid heart rate, and general discomfort for 8 to 10 hours. Febrile reactions are treated symptomatically.

be life-threatening, because the reaction can cause air passages to swell and prevent normal breathing.

Allergies are diagnosed by patient history, in which exposure to a particular substance is related to a reaction, and sometimes by the scratch test. In this test, suspected allergens are introduced into the uppermost layer of skin and the site is observed to note any reaction. (The diagnosis and treatment of several of these disorders are discussed in the appropriate books in this series: respiratory system—allergic rhinitis, asthma; dermatology—contact dermatitis.)

Acquired Immune Deficiency Syndrome (AIDS)

Acquired immune deficiency syndrome (AIDS) is one of the most deadly diseases to affect today's population. AIDS is caused by a bloodborne virus that attacks and eventually destroys the body's immune system. It is a sexually transmitted disease and primarily affects promiscuous homosexual and bisexual men, drug users who share hypodermic needles, and recipients of contaminated blood in transfusions. In addition, an infected mother can pass the virus to her fetus or during pregnancy or delivery.

While the vast majority of victims fall into one of the above categories, AIDS can be transmitted during vaginal intercourse and anyone participating in unprotected sex can be at risk. This is the case in Africa, where AIDS is primarily a heterosexual disease. (Study the discussion on sexually transmitted disease in the book on urology and the reproductive system in this series, for more information.)

AIDS was first identified in the United States in 1979. Apparently the syndrome, or pattern of illness, had not occurred previously. There were only 20 cases in 1979, but by 1991 there were 182,834 reported cases, and the numbers continue to increase.

At the present time, AIDS appears to occur in the following percentages: homosexual or bisexual males who have multiple sex partners (63 percent); users of intravenous drugs who share contaminated needles (19 percent); homosexual or bisexual intravenous drug users (7 percent); heterosexual men and women (4 percent); recipients of blood or blood products (3 percent); and patients with hemophilia who have received transfusions from pooled blood (1 percent).

The most common causative agent of AIDS is the **human immunodeficiency (IM yoo noh deh FISH en see) virus (HIV),** but recent studies have show that non-HIV agents can also transmit the disease. HIV has the ability to "take over" certain cells and interrupt their normal genetic functioning. Mainly, the T-4 lymphocytes of the body lose their ability to fight infection. HIV is a relatively weak virus. It is not transmitted through air or water, nor does it travel easily from person to person as other infections may. The virus is transmitted principally by direct intimate contact involving mucous membrane surfaces. The virus cannot penetrate skin but enters through natural body openings and wounds.

A newly infected person may not test positive for HIV for up to 1 year. A person with HIV may not develop AIDS for up to 10 years. Some HIV-positive people develop a mild form of AIDS known as **AIDS-related-complex (ARC),** which presents with mild clinical symptoms such as fever, weight loss, diarrhea, and swollen glands. About 25 percent of people with ARC develop full-blown AIDS within 3 years. Also, a substantial number of people have died from ARC without developing AIDS at all. At this time, all

victims of AIDS die, no cure is known and no vaccine is available to prevent it.

The symptoms of AIDS consist of recurrent, persistent, or rare infections, which normally would be quickly overcome by the immune system. The patient may have recurring fever, rapid weight loss, swollen lymph glands in the neck, underarms (axillae), and groin, fatigue, diarrhea, loss of appetite, and spots in the mouth. In later stages of the disease, infections become more severe and the patient is susceptible to rare diseases.

Two diseases that frequently occur in AIDS patients are **Kaposi's sarcoma (KAP oh seez sar KOH mah),** a type of cancer that appears as a skin abnormality, and *Pneumocystis carinii* **(new moh SIS tis kah RIH nee iye)** pneumonia, a lung infection caused by a parasite. The opportunistic infections that follow the syndrome may be treatable, but some do not respond. If the patient does recover from an infection, he or she remains susceptible to others that may not be treatable.

Health care professionals must exercise great precaution when handling blood or bodily secretions of AIDS patients. The best protection against AIDS exposure is consistent adherence to the universal precaution recommendations of the Centers for Diseases Control (CDC) (see Table 8). Several studies have been done to evaluate the risk of HIV transmission among health care workers, and the infection rate is very low when precautionary procedures are strictly observed. A few cases of health professionals developing antibodies against the virus after accidental cuts or needle pricks by contaminated instruments have been reported. Isolation of HIV has made possible the development of a blood test to detect the presence of antibodies indicating exposure to the disease. The test can be applied to stored blood,

Table 8: CDC Precautions Against AIDS Infection for Health Care Workers

I. Wear protective clothing.
   a) Wear gloves when touching blood or body fluids, mucous membranes, skin, soiled items, during venipuncture or other blood procedures. Change gloves after each patient.
   b) Wear a mask and protective eyewear or a face shield during procedures likely to generate droplets of blood or body fluid from the mouth, nose or eyes.
   c) Wear a gown or apron during procedures likely to splash blood or other body fluid.

II. Washing
Wash hands and other skin surfaces immediately and thoroughly if contaminated. Wash hands immediately after gloves are removed.

III. Prevent injuries
When handling, cleaning or disposing of needles, scalpel blades or other sharp instruments, be careful to take precautions not to be injured. Dispose properly.

IV. Use a ventilation device when performing mouth to mouth resuscitation.

V. Do not perform patient care if you have open skin lesions. Avoid handling patient-care equipment as well.

VI. Pregnant health care workers should be especially careful to adhere to universal precautions.

---

which reduces the risk of transmission by blood transfusions.

Researchers around the world are working toward designing a drug to effect a cure for AIDS. Currently, zidovudine, commonly called AZT, which originally was formulated as an anticancer drug, reduces the symptoms of AIDS and prolongs life by extending the symptom-free period between HIV infection and the onset of AIDS. It does not offer a cure, however.

Neutropenia

This term means a relative lack of neutrophils, which as we have seen is a type of white blood cell that combats bacterial infection. Other terms associated with low white blood cell counts are **granulocytopenia (GRAN yoo loh SYE toh PEE nee ah),** or a low level of all the granulocytes (neutrophils, basophils, and eosinophils) and **agranulocytosis (ah GRAN yoo loh sye TOH sis),** which means a total absence of granulocytes.

The condition makes patients highly susceptible to infection, which may be fatal depending on the extent of the condition.

Neutropenia (NYOO troh PEE nee ah) has a number of possible causes, ranging from inheritance to severe infection. Sometimes the cause is not known, and sometimes it is the result of taking certain drugs for another disease. Neutropenia is diagnosed on the basis of a white blood cell count, after which the physician must attempt to identify the cause.

First all drugs are stopped, and the physician looks for any signs or sites of infection. Bacterial infections are treated with appropriate antibiotics. Transfusions of white blood cells may be helpful, and splenectomy is useful in some cases. If the condition persists, the patient must be protected against infection as much as possible. If a low white cell count persists and is severe, the patient will eventually die from an infection.

Autoimmune Diseases

A number of diseases that until recently could not be classified by cause have been found to be the result of **autoimmune (AW toh im MYOON) diseases.** In these diseases, the immune system reacts against a part of the body itself, for no apparent reason. The plasma cells generate antibodies that continue an inflammatory process indefinitely, destroy certain blood cells, or otherwise threaten normal body functions. Some examples of autoimmune diseases:

- **Rheumatoid arthritis (ROO mah toyd ar THRYE tis),** which causes inflammation in one or more joints (discussed more fully in the orthopedics book of this series);
- **Hashimoto's (HASH ih MOH tohz) disease,** in which the immune system gradually destroys the thyroid gland;
- **Myasthenia gravis (MYE as THEE nee ah GRAY vis),** which affects the transmission of nerve impulses to certain muscles; and
- **Polymyositis (POL ee MYE oh SYE tis),** in which muscles in the shoulders and hips become inflamed;
- **Systemic lupus erythematosus (LOO pus er ih THEE mah TOH sis),** or SLE, is a serious autoimmune disease which causes inflammation of the connective tissue. It affects the skin and causes deterioration of all collagenous connective tissue. It also affects the glomeruli of the kidneys, causing an elevation in the excretion of albumin as well as blood and casts. The lining of the heart can also be affected, deteriorating as the disease progresses. Systemic lupus can have a sudden onset or may begin slowly, usually in young women. The patient may complain of rashes, especially a macular butterfly redness on the face. The skin becomes overly sensitive to sunlight. There may also be joint and muscle pains or swollen lymph nodes. The disease often involves periods of remission and periods of exacerbation. Corticosteroids are given to control the symptoms. Systemic lupus erythematosus may be fatal, particularly if kidney or heart failure develops. Since there is a decreased number of leukocytes there may also be a susceptibility to opportunistic infections, such as pneumonia.

In general, autoimmune diseases are treated by giving immunosuppressive drugs and/or steroids to combat the abnormal antibodies. Other forms of treatment are aimed at relieving the symptoms. (These diseases are discussed in more detail in the books in this series that deal with the affected systems.)

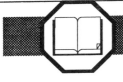 **STOP AND REVIEW**

Fill in the blanks

1. Diseases of the lymphatic and immune systems can affect the entire body because _____ .

2. Treatment of immune disease usually requires _____ of the patient, or protection of the patient against _____ .

3. Swollen lymph nodes usually result from mild infections in _____ .

(continued next page)

STOP AND REVIEW

Short answers

4. Name two common infections of the lymph nodes and list their treatment.

   a. _____

   b. _____

5. Identify two tests used to diagnose lymphadenopathy.

   a. _____

   b. _____

6. List three effects of hypersplenism.

   a. _____

   b. _____

   c. _____

7. Name three causes of immunodeficiencies.

   a. _____

   b. _____

   c. _____

8. Current research indicates that AIDS is transmitted by what two main behaviors?

   a. _____

   b. _____

9. Describe the disposal of blood or body fluids from AIDS patients. _____
   _____

10. Identify two autoimmune diseases.

    a. _____

    b. _____

Fill in the blanks

11. Infection from opportunistic pathogens such as _____ and
    _____ is characteristic of AIDS.

12. _____ is a term meaning relative lack of neutrophils.

13. Because they appear on lymphatic tissue, lymphomas can be located _____ .

14. Hodgkin's disease is distinguished from other kinds of lymphomas by the presence of
    _____ .

15. In autoimmune disorders, _____ cells generate antibodies that
    function against some part of the body itself.

A

AIDS See Acquired immune deficiency syndrome.

Abscess A collection of pus in an acute or chronic, localized infection, usually associated with tissue destruction and swelling.

Acid-base balance A state of equilibrium between acidity and alkalinity of body fluids: the normal pH range of the blood is 7.35–7.45 pH (slightly alkaline, or base).

Acidosis Accumulation of acid or depletion of alkaline bicarbonate of the blood; untreated, it causes drowsiness, coma, eventually death.

Acquired immune deficiency syndrome (AIDS) Pattern of illnesses that is caused by the human immunodeficiency virus (HIV); an excess of one type of T-cell inhibits the manufacture of antibodies against infection; transmitted by sexual contact or by contact with the blood of an infected person.

Acquired immunity Resistance to disease resulting from exposure to the causative pathogen; may be active, naturally acquired immunity from having had the disease, or artificial passive immunity having acquired antibodies from a person with active immunity; artificial active immunity results from intentional vaccination with weakened pathogens.

Activated lymphocyte One that has responded immunologically after exposure to an antigen.

Active immunity Acquired immunity caused by the presence of antibodies that formed in response to an antigen.

Acute lymphocytic leukemia Neoplastic disorder most often found in children, in which cancerous lymphocytes, primarily immature forms, enter the bloodstream and damage the liver, spleen, bone marrow, and central nervous system. Production of blood cells in the bone marrow is disrupted.

Acute myelogenous leukemia Neoplastic disorder in which immature granulocytes in the bone marrow multiply instead of maturing, disrupting production of other blood cells, and later enter the bloodstream, damaging such organs as the liver and spleen.

Acute transformation A phase in chronic myelogenous leukemia when treatment is no longer effective and the disease resembles acute leukemia, usually followed by progressively shorter remissions and finally death.

Afferent lymphatic vessel Collecting vessel entering the lymph nodes, bringing in foreign substances to be filtered out.

Agglutination Clumping together, as of red blood cells when an antigen is present.

Agranulocytosis Total absence of granulocytes in the blood.

AIDS related complex (ARC) Mild form of acquired immune deficiency syndrome (AIDS), which produces mild clinical symptoms such as fever, weight loss, diarrhea, and swollen glands.

Albumin The most plentiful of the plasma proteins. Formed in the liver, its major function is to attract water from the interstitial fluid into the blood; it also combines with amino acids, fatty acids, hormones, and minerals to keep them from being filtered out of the blood.

Alkalosis Accumulation of base or loss of acid in the blood or a decrease in H+ ions; untreated, it causes overstimulation of the CNS and of the muscles.

Allergen Antigen that causes a hypersensitivity reaction only in certain individuals, being harmless to others.

Allergy A state of abnormal and individual hypersensitivity in which re-exposure to an allergen causes a reaction such as inflammation of the respiratory system.

Alpha globulin See Globulin.

Anaphylaxis Unusual or extreme allergic reaction, which can be fatal.

Anemia Inadequate number of erythrocytes in the blood, or inadequate quantity of hemoglobin in the erythrocytes.

Anisocytosis Abnormal variations in sizes of red blood cells.

Antibody Specific immunoglobulin substance produced by plasma cells formed from B-cells in response to the presence of a specific antigen.

Antibody-mediated immunity See Humoral immunity.

Anticoagulant Substance that prevents or restricts blood clotting.

Antigen Specific substance, such as a virus, a toxin, a foreign protein, a grain of pollen, that incites B-cells to produce plasma cells that then produce antibodies against the substance, as well as memory cells that will respond to that substance at a later time by producing more antibodies.

Antihemophilic factor See Factor VIII.

Antiserum (pl. antisera) Commercially prepared pure suspension of antibodies that will react only with a specific antigen.

Antithrombin Substance that opposes the action of thrombin in the clotting process, thus limiting coagulation.

Aplastic anemia Disorder in which the bone marrow reduces production of all blood cells.

Appendectomy   Surgical removal of the appendix.

Appendicitis   An inflammation of the appendix.

Arrhythmias   Any abnormal heart rhythm.

Autoimmune disease   Immunologic reaction in which the body's own cells or antibodies turn against some part of the body itself. For example, plasma cells generate antibodies that continue the inflammatory process indefinitely, destroy certain blood cells, or otherwise threaten normal body functions. Rheumatoid arthritis and myasthenia gravis are examples.

Axillary nodes   Lymph nodes located in the armpits (axillae).

B

Bacteriolysis   Breaking down or dissolution of bacterial cells.

Band cell   Immature neutrophil with a horseshoe-shaped nucleus.

Basophil   Granular leukocyte with an S-shaped, bilobed nucleus and cytoplasmic granules that stain dark purple with basic dyes or bluish-black with Wright's stain. Basophils contain the anticoagulant heparin; their function is unknown.

Basophilic stippling   Blue network appearing on abnormal red blood cells stained with basic dye.

B-cells   See Lymphocytes.

Beta globulin   See Globulin.

Bleeding time test   Test in which the time required for a small incision to stop bleeding is compared to a known standard. The test can be helpful in determining platelet functioning and vasoconstriction.

Blood clot   Product of the coagulation process, comprised of platelets and fibrin.

Blood group   One of four major groups or types of blood, differentiated by the type of antigens appearing on the red blood cells and the antibodies appearing in the blood plasma. The groups are A, B, AB, and O.

B-lymphocytes   See Lymphocytes.

Biconcave disk   Disk that has two concave (or indented) surfaces.

Bile   Fluid secreted by the liver through the bile ducts and into the small intestine.

Bilirubin   A red bile pigment formed from hemoglobin during the normal or abnormal destruction of erythrocytes by the reticuloendothelial system.

Blood   The "circulating tissue" of the body made up of plasma and formed elements.

Bone marrow transplantation   Experimental treatment of certain blood diseases by replacing diseased marrow with carefully matched donated marrow.

Brachiocephalic veins   Two veins that drain lymph from the head, neck, and upper extremities.

Buffers   A mixture of an acid and a base which, when present in a solution, reduces any changes in the pH that might otherwise occur.

C

Cabot ring   Blue ring that appears in certain red blood cells stained with a polychromatic stain.

Cell-mediated immunity   Body defense, provided by specifically sensitized T-cells (lymphocytes) which attack specific antigens.

Cervical nodes   Lymph nodes located in the neck.

Chronic lymphocytic leukemia   Overproduction of lymphocytes most often found in adults, with symptoms like those of acute lymphocytic leukemia.

Chronic myelogenous leukemia   Chronic form of acute myelogenous leukemia that causes mature granulocytes to multiply to 20–40 times the normal number, disrupting production of other blood cells, damaging the spleen and liver, and decreasing protection against infection because the cancerous granulocytes are not effective against bacteria.

Chyle   A white or pale yellow fluid taken up by the lymphatics from the intestine during digestion; it is carried into the circulation.

Cisterna chyli   Widened or dilated part of the thoracic duct at its origin in the lumbar region that holds chyle (lymph permeated with fat).

Clotting mechanism   See Coagulation.

Coagulation   Formation of blood clots in a complex chemical process. Platelets adhere to a tear, rough place, or deposit on a blood vessel and release chemicals (platelet factors) that accelerate coagulation and constrict the surrounding blood vessels. Prothrombin in the plasma reacts with the platelet factors and with calcium to produce thrombin, which reacts with fibrinogen to produce fibrin. Fibrin, fine thread-like fibers, forms a net that traps red blood cells and holds platelets in place at the site, forming a clot.

Coagulation test   Test in which clotting time of a sample is compared to a known standard for normal blood.

Complement   A complex series of enzymatic proteins in normal serum that interact with the antibody-antigen complex, producing lysis.

Complex   In the immune system, a specific antibody-antigen combination.

Corpuscle   Literally "little body"; blood cell.

Crenated red cell   Red blood cell that shrinks and has abnormal notched, spiny edges.

Cytoplasm   Interior of the cell.

Cytotoxic substance   Substance released by T-cells that destroys antigen products directly.

D

Daughter cells Cells produced by the stem cells which differentiate into primitive forms of the various blood cells.

Differential blood cell count Blood test done to determine the number of each type of white blood cells present, and whether they are normal and mature.

Diluent Making watery by diluting; an agent that dilutes.

E

ESR See Erythrocyte sedimentation rate.

Efferent lymphatic vessel Vessel leaving the lymph nodes, carrying out the filtered lymph. Efferent vessels join to form larger vessels that lead to either the thoracic duct or the right lymphatic duct.

Eosinophil Granular leukocyte usually with a bilobed nucleus whose cytoplasmic round granules stain orange with acid dyes (eosins) or red with Wright's stain. Their function is not fully established, but their number increases during allergic reactions and parasitic infections.

Erythroblast Nucleated precursor of erythrocyte.

Erythroblastosis fetalis Agglutination of the fetal blood cells that results from Rh incompatibility between mother and fetus.

Erythrocyte Red blood cell, transporter of oxygen to the cells and carbon dioxide to the lungs. Mature erythrocytes lack nuclei; they are flexible biconcave disks capable of passing through the arterioles and venules of the circulatory system. See also Reticulocyte.

Erythrocyte sedimentation rate (ESR) Test employing the extent and rate at which red blood cells settle as a measure for detecting inflammation (the settling rate increases in inflammatory diseases).

Erythropoiesis Process of formation of erythrocytes or red blood cells from stem cells in the red bone marrow.

F

Factor Vitamins or other essential element, especially in blood.

Factor VIII A contributing cause of blood clotting, its deficiency is linked with hemophilia; also called antihemophilic factor.

Fibrin Insoluble, thread-like fibers produced by the reaction of thrombin and fibrinogen in the coagulation process.

Fibrinogen Plasma protein that by the action of thrombin is converted to fibrin in the clotting process.

Fibrinolysin Proteolytic enzyme in the blood that dissolves fibrin and thus breaks down a blood clot.

Fibrinolysis Dissolution or destruction of fibrin (in blood clots) by the blood enzyme fibrinolysin.

Folic acid One of the B complex vitamins, involved in the synthesis of amino acids and DNA.

Folic acid-deficiency anemia Disorder similar to iron-deficiency anemia, except that the missing ingredient is folic acid. Common in pregnancy.

Formed elements See Blood cells.

G

G6-P-D deficiency See Glucose-6-phosphate-dehydrogenase deficiency.

Gamma globulin See Globulin.

Globulin A general term for proteins that are insoluble in water but soluble in saline solutions; all plasma proteins except albumin. Globulins include alpha, beta, and gamma globulins. The first two combine with proteins to carry them to other parts of the body; gamma globulin contains antibodies and is part of the immune system.

Glucose-6-phosphate-dehydrogenase deficiency (G6-P-D deficiency) Inherited blood disorder caused by deficiency or lack of an enzyme, G6-P-D, in erythrocytes. Patients with this disorder (usually males, because it is sex-linked) may develop hemolytic anemia in response to certain infections, drugs, or eating certain foods. The disorder is found most often in males of African or Mediterranean descent.

Gram-negative bacteria Bacteria that lose color when responding to Gram's stain; they have a more complex cell wall than gram-positive bacteria.

Granular leukocytes See Leukocyte.

Granulocytopenia Depressed production of granulocytes leaving the body defenseless against bacterial invasion.

H

Hashimoto's desease An autoimmune disorder thought to be the most common cause of primary hypothyroidism; autoantibodies to thyroglobin are characteristic of the disease; also called autoimmune thyoiditis.

Helper T-cell Form of T-cell that helps B-cells to recognize certain antigens.

Hemacytometer Device used to count blood corpuscles.

Hematocrit The volume percentage of erythrocytes in whole blood.

Hematopoiesis Formation and development of blood cells from primitive stem cells, mostly in the red bone marrow, but also in the lymphatic system and lungs. The stem cells replicate by mitosis, differentiate into early forms of various cells, pass through several stages of growth, and at maturity are released into the bloodstream.

Hematopoietic stem cell Primitive cell from which blood cells develop.

Hemoglobin The red protein in erythrocytes responsible for oxygen and carbon dioxide transportation.

Hemolysis The breaking down or rupture of red blood cells releasing hemoglobin into the plasma.

Hemolytic anemia Anemia caused by shortened survival of mature erythrocytes and inability of the bone marrow to compensate for their decreased life span. In some cases, due to a hereditary abnormality in the blood.

Hemophilia A condition of impaired coagulability of the blood with a strong tendency to bleed. The individual (usually male, because hemophilia is sex-linked) has a deficiency of the protein clotting Factor VIII.

Heparin An acid mucopolysaccharide present in basophils, the lungs, liver, and other tissues, which has anticoagulant properties.

Hepatitis Liver inflammation.

Hereditary spherocytosis Inherited congenital form of hemolytic anemia in which red blood cells are spherical and more fragile than normal. Jaundice and enlarged spleen are additional characteristics.

Histamine Chemical mediator of the inflammatory response, which dilates capillaries, contracts smooth muscles, increases gastric secretion, and increases the heart rate.

Hodgkin's disease A neoplastic disease of the primary lymph nodes characterized by painless, progressive enlargement of the lymph nodes, spleen, and lymphoid tissues generally. Also called malignant granuloma, lymphogranuloma.

Howell-Jolly body Small, round granules, probably remnants of nuclei, seen in red blood cells and found in various anemias and after splenectomy.

Human immunodeficiency virus (HIV) Virus responsible for acquired immune deficiency syndrome (AIDS).

Humoral immunity Body defense to specific substances called antigens, provided by antibodies produced by plasma cells that develop from lymphocytes called B-cells.

Hypersplenism Disorder in which the spleen becomes hyperactive, enlarges, and destroys excessive numbers of all types of blood cells.

Hypochromia Abnormally pale red blood cells, caused by reduced hemoglobin content.

Hypothalamus A portion of the brain lying beneath the thalamus which functions as part of the autonomic nervous system.

I

IgA Serum and secretor immunoglobulins found in nonvascular fluids such as bile, mucus, saliva, and tears; works with the nonspecific immune system to protect mucous membranes by keeping microorganisms from attaching to epithelial cells. They have antiviral properties.

IgD Immunoglobulin found in trace quantities (about 3 mg/dl) in the serum; it serves as a B-cell surface receptor.

IgE Immunoglobulin that binds with mucous membrane and skin cells which become sensitized to allergens to cause the cells to release histamine and other substances in allergic reactions.

IgG Most prevalent of the immunoglobulins, and the one that can cross the placenta during pregnancy, providing the fetus with passive immunity. It serves as an antibody in the humoral response and is involved in activating the complement system and in opsonization.

IgM Immunoglobulin that also activates the complement system to destroy foreign antigens such as foreign tissue in transplanted organs.

Iatrogenic disease Disease resulting from treatment by a physician or surgeon.

Immune response The reaction to and interaction with substances interpreted by the body as foreign; the result is humoral and cellular immunity.

Immunization Introduction of a weak or diluted form of an antigen into the body being rendered immune, causing a humoral immune system response: production of plasma cells, antibodies, and memory cells.

Immunodeficiency Deficiency of a humoral antibody or lymphoid cell immune response, causing susceptibility to certain types of infection.

Immunoglobulins Proteins found in blood plasma that function as antibodies. The five classes of immunoglobulins of the humoral immune response are IgG, IgA, IgM, IgD, and IgE. They are synthesized by lymphocytes and plasma cells.

Incubation period Time between exposure to disease and start of symptoms during which the infectious agent builds up to a level at which plasma cells start to make antibodies, and reactions occur, causing such symptoms as fever.

Inflammatory response Body's response to injury in which the nonspecific internal defense systems immediately go into action.

Inguinal nodes Lymph nodes located in the groin.

Interferon A glycoprotein released by cells invaded by viruses. It stimulates noninfected cells to synthesize another antiviral protein.

Interstitial fluid Fluid between tissues.

Intrinsic factor A glycoprotein synthesized in the intestinal tract that facilitates vitamin B_{12} absorption.

Iron-deficiency anemia Anemia characterized by low or absent iron stores, low serum iron concentration, low hemoglobin, and hypochromic, microcytic red blood corpuscles.

K

Kaposi's sarcoma Type of cancer that appears as a skin abnormality, especially in patients with AIDS.

Killer macrophages Monocytes that have been converted by lymphokines which destroy all surrounding cells, whether foreign or not.

Killer T-cell An activated, sensitized T-cell which migrates to the site of invasion. It attaches to the antigen and releases four substances: cytotoxic substances which destroy antigen directly; transfer factor, which causes nonsensitized lymphocytes at the invasion site to resemble the sensitized T-cell; macrophage chemotactic factor, which attracts macrophages to the site of invasion; and macrophage activating factor, which increases the phagocytic activity of macrophages.

Kinins Chemical mediator of the inflammatory response, which causes vasodilation, increases permeability, decreases blood pressure, and causes smooth muscle contraction.

L

Leukemia A malignant disease of the blood-forming organs characterized by a rapid and abnormal increase in the number of white blood cells.

Leukocyte White blood cell; may be granular or nongranular (depending on presence or absence of granules in the cytoplasm); granular leukocytes include neutrophils, eosinophils, and basophils; nongranular leukocytes are lymphocytes and monocytes. Leukocytes function as part of the immune system, leaving the blood vessels to enter the interstitial fluid and phagocytose foreign material. See also under names of individual leukocytes.

Leukopenia Reduced number of leukocytes in the blood.

Lingual tonsils See Tonsils.

Lymph Transparent fluid, collected from all body tissues and returned to the blood via the lymphatic system; its composition is 95% water and similar to blood plasma.

Lymph capillary The smallest of the lymph vessels.

Lymph node Larger oval-shaped collections of lymphatic tissue found in clusters along the lymphatic vessels. They are the main source of lymphocytes in the peripheral blood. The major clusters of lymph nodes are the cervical, submaxillary, axillary, and inguinal nodes.

Lymph nodule Small collection of lymphatic tissue found in areas of the body regularly exposed to outside contamination, such as the lining of the digestive system, the respiratory system, and the urinary tract.

Lymphadenitis Swollen glands, an accumulation of large numbers of bacteria or viruses in lymph nodes, inflaming them.

Lymphadenopathy Disease of the lymph nodes.

Lymphatic system Network of vessels, together with lymph nodes, ducts, the spleen, and the thymus, which circulates the fluid lymph, filtering toxins, sediment, and waste products, manufacturing lymphocytes and monocytes, destroying worn-out or defective red blood cells, and carrying fat from the intestines to the blood. The lymphatic system eventually drains into the bloodstream.

Lymphoblast The immature, nucleolated precursor of the mature lymphocyte.

Lymphocyte Nongranular leukocyte, chiefly a product of the lymphoid tissue, that appears as undifferentiated cells; B-cells that form antibodies; or T-cells that function in the lymphatic system. Also see under names of individual lymphocytes.

Lymphokine A general term denoting soluble protein mediators released by sensitized lymphocytes and believed to play a role in macrophage activation, lymphocyte transformation, and cell-mediated immunity.

Lymphoma Any neoplastic disorder of lymphoid tissue, including Hodgkin's disease.

Lyse To break up or disintegrate.

Lysis The breakup or disintegration of a substance, such as lysis of fibrin which breaks up a blood clot.

M

Macrocytosis A condition of larger-than-normal red blood cells in a specimen. A form of anisocytosis. Also called microcythemia.

Macrohematocrit method Method of measuring hematocrit that requires more blood and uses a larger Wintrobe tube than the microhematocrit method.

Macrophage Large mononuclear cells that are highly phagocytic.

Macrophage activating factor (MAF) Substance released by T-cells that increases the phagocytic activity of macrophages.

Macrophage chemotactic factor Substance released by T-cells that attracts additional macrophages to an invasion site.

Marker See Antigen.

Mast cells Cells in loose connective tissue along blood vessels which produce heparin.

Matrix The intercellular substance of a tissue, such as bone matrix, or the tissue from which a structure develops, such as hair or nail matrix.

Megakaryocytes A large cell with a multilobulated nucleus that gives rise to blood platelets.

Memory cells Cells derived from B-cells which arise when an antigen enters the body; they are programmed to release antibodies when the same antigen reappears.

Memory T-cell A T-cell activated by the thymus to recognize the original invading antigen and initiate a swift antibody reaction.

Metastatic cancer Cancer that migrates from one area to another that is not directly connected to the original area.

Microcytosis Anisocytosis in which many red blood cells are smaller than normal. Also called microcythemia.

Microhematocrit A measurement of the percentage

of total blood volume occupied by red blood cells using only a small amount of blood in a test tube; see Hematocrit.

Mitosis The process of cell reproduction in which cells replicate constantly by dividing, producing daughter cells, which differentiate into primitive forms of the various blood cells.

Monocyte Largest of the leukocytes; nongranular leukocyte with an ovoid or kidney-shaped nucleus. Monocytes are derived from the bone marrow, circulate in the blood for 1 day, migrate to tissues such as the lung and liver, and then develop into macrophages.

Monokines Proteins secreted by macrophages which stimulate T-cell reproduction and cause fever.

Multiple myeloma Malignant neoplastic disease of plasma cells. The plasma cell proliferation disrupts production of other cells in the bone marrow, causing destruction of the bone. Antibody production, the kidneys, and the nervous system are also affected.

Myasthenia gravis A chronic progressive muscular weakness that usually begins in the face and throat accompanied by atrophy, an autoimmune disorder.

Myeloblast An immature cell of the granulocytic series occurring in bone marrow; matures into a myelocyte.

Myelocyte A young cell of the granulocytic series found in bone marrow but not circulating in the blood; matures into a metamyelocyte.

N

Neutropenia Diminished number of neutrophils in the blood, making patients very susceptible to infections.

Neutrophil Granular leukocyte having a nucleus with three to five lobes and cytoplasmic granules that stain pruplish blue with Wright's stain. The most numerous of all leukocytes. They fight bacterial infections. Also called polymorphonuclear leukocytes.

Nongranular leukocytes See Leukocyte.

Nonspecific immune response Generalized reactions of several body systems against all types of foreign materials.

Nonspecific immuune system The wide variety of body reactionsagainst a wide range of pathogens. White blood cells and lymphatic system responses to all foreign substances; also includes secretions of the mucous membranes, sweat grands, sebaceous glands, and lacrimal glands, which move potentially harmful substances out of or off of the body.

O

Opsonization Preparation of foreign cells and bacteria for phagocytosis by cells in the immune system.

Ovalocytosis Condition in which red blood cells are oval in shape rather than round disks. Also called elliptocytosis.

P

Palatine tonsils See Tonsils.

Passive immunity Temporary protection provided by the mother's antibodies to the infant, or by injections of antibodies, such as tetanus or diphtheria, to reinforce the exposed patient's immune system.

Pernicious anemia Incurable form of vitamin B$_{12}$ deficiency in which the gastric mucous membrane does not produce intrinsic factor, necessary for the absorption of the vitamin in the stomach and essential to the formation of erythrocytes.

pH Symbol for the relative acidity or alkalinity of a solution.

Phagocytosis The engulfing of foreign material, microorganisms, or other cells in the body by phagocytes.

Pharyngeal tonsils See Tonsils.

Plasma Pale yellow liquid composed of approximately 90% water and 10% solutes; the fluid component of blood in which corpuscles are suspended.

Plasma proteins The predominant solutes in blood plasma; include albumin, fibrinogen, and globulins.

Platelet See Thrombocyte.

Platelet count Test in which mature red blood cells are destroyed by a diluent; the sample is then put into a hemacytometer or a machine for counting the remaining cells (including white blood cells, platelets, and immature red cells).

Platelet factor Factors important in hemostasis, which are contained in or attached to the platelets.

Pneumocystis carinii An organism that causes a pneumonia commonly found in AIDS patients.

Poikilocytosis A condition of abnormally shaped erythrocytes in the blood.

Polycythemia Benign neoplastic disease in which the bone marrow overproduces normal blood cells. The form of the disorder called polycythemia vera causes overproduction of all blood cells; the form called secondary polycythemia causes overproduction of erythrocytes only.

Polycythemia vera See Polycythemia.

Polychromatophilia Affinity for many stains. A condition in which red blood cells stain with various blue shades and pink tinges.

Polymorphonuclear leukocytes See Neutrophils.

Polymyositis Autoimmune disease in which shoulder and hip muscles become inflamed.

Polys See Neutrophils.

Precipitation The act of causing solid particles in solution to settle.

Primordial stem cell See Hematopoietic stem cell.

Prostaglandin Chemical mediator of the inflammatory response, which decreases blood pressure, and regulates stomach acid secretion, temperature, and platelet aggregation.

Prothrombin Plasma glycoprotein that is converted to thrombin by extrinsic thromboplastin during the second stage of blood clotting. Test to measure the activity of clotting factors V, VII, X, prothrombin, and fibrinogen.

Prothrombin time test Test in which an anticoagulant preventing conversion of prothrombin to thrombin is added to a blood sample; calcium and thromboplastin are then added. The time required for these additives to clot the specimen is compared to the normal time for coagulation, which is 12 to 15 seconds.

Pus Liquid composed of dead white blood cells; the product of infection or inflammation.

R

Reed-Sternberg cell A characteristic cell found in affected tissue in Hodgkin's disease.

Remission A period during which the symptoms of a disease disappear and the body resumes normal function.

Rheumatoid arthritis An autoimmune disorder characterized by inflammation of one or more joints.

Rh factor Protein appearing in the red blood cells of certain individuals. Such persons (85% of whites) are Rh-positive, persons whose blood does not contain the factor are Rh-negative. A mother with Rh-negative blood can build up antibodies to Rh-positive blood of a fetus late in a first pregnancy; in later Rh-positive pregnancies antibodies in the mother's blood can cross the placenta into the fetal blood and cause agglutination (erythroblastosis fetalis), which is fatal if not treated.

Rh-negative See Rh factor.

Rh-positive See Rh factor.

Rho-GAM Drug that prevents formation of antibodies against the Rh-factor by binding (tying up) the fetal Rh + antigens so that the mother's system will respond with production of anti-Rh antibodies; it is given to Rh-negative mothers when Rh-positive babies are delivered.

Red blood cell count Test in which a diluent preserves red blood cells for counting in a hemacytometer.

Reticulocyte Erythrocyte in the stage just before maturity; shows basophilic reticulum when stained. The percentage of reticulocytes in the circulation can be an indication of disease.

Reticulocyte count Test in which the percentage of reticulocytes compared to mature erythrocytes in a specimen is calculated, to determine whether the bone marrow is producing red cells at a normal rate.

Reticuloendothelial cell Part of the immune system; cells lining the blood vessels, liver, spleen, lungs, and bone marrow that phagocytose worn-out red blood cells, store fatty materials, and metabolize iron and pigment. Some of the cells are motile.

Right lymphatic duct Smaller of the two ducts in the lymphatic system, draining vessels from the upper right half of the body and emptying into the right brachiocephalic vein.

S

Septicemia Blood poisoning, systemic disease associated with the presence and persistence of pathogenic microorganisms or their toxins in the blood.

Serum Clear liquid resulting after the fibrin clot and blood cells have been separated out.

Sickle cell anemia Inherited disorder in which an abnormal form of hemoglobin is produced; erythrocytes with this hemoglobin wear out faster than normal and become deformed (sickle-shaped). Sickle cells do not pass through small blood vessels as easily as normal cells, causing blocked capillaries and lack of oxygen. An individual with two sickle cell genes will have the disorder. See also Sickle cell trait.

Sickle cell trait Possession of only one sickle cell gene. Such an individual will not have sickle cell anemia, but has the capability of passing the gene on to offspring.

Sinuses Channels that surround the compartments in which hematopoietic cells make lymphocytes.

Specific immune response Reactions against specific diseases by destroying or deactivating invading antigens with the antibodies.

Spectrophotometer Device that measures the color intensity of whole blood plasma or serum that has been mixed with a reagent.

Spectrophotometry The use of an apparatus for determining the quantity of coloring matter in a solution by measurement of transmitted light.

Spherocytosis Condition in which red blood cells are small, globular, and hemoglobinated.

Spleen A large gland-like ductless organ made up of lymphatic tissue, connective tissue, and smooth muscle fibers. Part of the lymphatic system, the spleen produces lymphocytes (in the white splenic pulp) and is the largest producer of reticuloendothelial cells, which destroy defective red blood cells and foreign particles (in the red splenic pulp). It also extracts iron and bilirubin from red blood cells; the first is sent to the liver and the second is eliminated in the bile.

Splenectomy Surgical removal of the spleen, used in treatment of certain blood diseases.

Splenic pulp A framework within the spleen divided into red and white splenic pulp; splenic pulp produces lymphocytes; blood leaves the vessels and flows through the red splenic pulp where defective and foreign material are filtered out and destroyed.

Submaxillary nodes Lymph nodes located in the floor of the mouth.

Suppressor T-cell Suppressor T-cells can inhibit the secretion of injurious substances by killer T-cells and inhibit the development of B-cells into antibody-producing plasma cells.

Swollen glands   See Lymphadenitis.

Systemic lupus erythematosus   An autoimmune disease that causes progressive inflammation of the connective tissue.

T

T-cells   See Lymphocytes.

Thalassemia   A heterogeneous group of hereditary hemolytic anemias marked by decreased rate of synthesis of one or more hemoglobin polypeptide chains.

Thoracic duct   Larger of the two ducts in the lymphatic system; lymph vessels from the left side of the head, neck, and chest, the left upper extremity, and the entire body below the ribs drain into the thoracic duct.

Thrombin   Enzyme product of the reaction of prothrombin with platelet factors and calcium in the bloodstream during the coagulation process. Thrombin catalyzes the conversion of fibrinogen to fibrin.

Thrombocyte   (also called platelet) Formed element in the blood, irregularly shaped fragments of larger cells (megakaryocytes) that are found in the bone marrow. Platelets help prevent blood loss by adhering to damaged blood vessels and forming plugs.

Thrombocytopenia   Disorder in which the number of platelets in the blood is decreased. Can be a symptom of leukemia or excessive blood loss. Most common in those of African, Italian, Greek, Arabian, and Indian descent.

Thymus   Ductless gland-like body of lymphatic tissue lying in the upper mediastinum beneath the sternum that programs lymphocytes to become T-cells; important in cell-mediated immunity. The thymus is largest in puberty, and shrinks afterward. ·

T-lymphocytes   See Lymphocytes.

Thalassemia major   See Thalassemia.

Thromboplastin   Substance with coagulant activity.

Tonsillectomy   Surgical removal of the tonsils.

Tonsillitis   An inflammation of the palatine or pharyngeal tonsils, which are a collection of lymphoid tissue.

Tonsils   Clusters of lymphatic tissue in three areas: pharyngeal, lingual, and palatine (around the apex (top) of the pharynx). These tissues help filter circulating lymph of bacteria and other foreign material.

Toxin   A poisonous substance; may be formed as part of a cell or as an extracellular product during metabolism and growth of an organism.

Transfer factor   Substance released by T-cells that causes nonsensitized lymphocytes to act like sensitized T-cells.

Transfusion   Process of replacing lost blood with donated blood that has been carefully matched, or introduction of donated blood components, such as red cells, platelets, whole plasma, or plasma components.

Transfusion reaction   The clumping or agglutination hemolysis of red blood cells and release of cellular elements into the serum when blood groups are incompatible.

U

Universal donor   Blood Type O, which has no hostile antigens on the red cells, and can thus (theoretically) be accepted by persons of any other blood type.

Universal recipient   Blood Type AB, which has no antibodies in the blood plasma to cause agglutination when combined with other blood types. However, factors other than antigens and antibodies can cause transfusion reactions.

V

Vaccination   See Immunization.

Vaccine   Dead or very weakened antigens for a specific disease injected into the body to develop immunity against that particular antigen.

Vitamin B$_{12}$ Water-soluble vitamin that is essential to red blood cell production.

Vitamin B$_{12}$-deficiency anemia   Disorder similar to iron-deficiency anemia, except that the missing ingredient is vitamin B$_{12}$ which is needed in the production of hemoglobin and the formation of erythrocytes. Found in those who do not eat a balanced diet; may also be iatrogenic in patients who have had digestive tract surgery.

W

White blood cell count   A test in which mature red blood cells are destroyed by a diluent; the sample is then put into a hemacytometer for counting the remaining cells (including white blood cells, platelets, and immature red cells).